"Everyone who rides wants to go faster—that's true whether you compete, are out to get fit and lose weight, or simply want to have more fun on your bike. This book shows you how to tune your body, your bike, and even your mind to reach your goal that much sooner."

—Peter Flax, editor in chief, Bicycling *magazine*

"Selene melds together the best and most recent science of training and nutrition to bring you practical aspects that really work! I am looking to get fast again (post baby); the proven science and sound advice Selene offers is the fast track to speed!"

—Stacy T. Sims, PhD, CISSN, chief research officer for Osmo Nutrition

"*Get Fast!* delivers! This is a no-BS compendium of highly effective training science and proven methodology. Selene Yeager gets on with the point quickly and gives the reader the tools to improve today with the inside skinny on the tricks of pros and the nuggets of cutting edge sports science without all the fluff. This entertaining and well thought-out book is certain to impact your performance immediately. I wish there was a book like this when I started racing!"

—Jeremiah Bishop, two-time USA National Mountain Bike Champion

"I've never been accused of being fast, but after reading Selene's book and acting on the excellent advice she offers, I just may turn some heads."

—Steve Madden, general manager of Sports on Earth
and former editor in chief of Bicycling magazine

"In 25 years of being an athlete, I've picked up my fair share of fitness books looking for inspiration and the holy grail of performance. *Get Fast!* is the first training book I've read cover to cover. True to her style, Selene Yeager, the Fit Chick, gets the info to you quickly by distilling a sea of training information into simple, effective nuggets that will benefit any athlete. She covers all of the pieces of the performance pie including mental training, equipment, flexibility, and more. Her easy-to-implement strategies are backed up by science and, more importantly, her own personal experience. *Get Fast!* is by far the most complete, realistic, and simple compilation of the best performance advice out there. Need proof that the *Get Fast!* strategies work? Just line up with Selene and watch as she rides away from you!"

—Rebecca Rusch, three-time World Champion Endurance Mountain Biker, four-time
Leadville 100 Winner, motivational speaker, and Gold Rusch tour manager

GET FAST!

A Complete Guide to Gaining Speed
Wherever You Ride

SELENE YEAGER

RODALE.

© 2013 by Rodale Inc.

Photographs (Illustrations) © 2013 by Rodale Inc.

Rodale books may be purchased for business or promotional use or for special sales. For information, please write to:

Special Markets Department, Rodale, Inc., 733 Third Avenue, New York, NY 10017

Bicycling is a registered trademark of Rodale Inc.

Printed in the United States of America

Rodale Inc. makes every effort to use acid-free ♾, recycled paper ♻.

Book design by Christina Gaugler

Photographs by Mitch Mandel

Library of Congress Cataloging-in-Publication Data is on file with the publisher.

ISBN 978-1-60961-831-5   paperback

Distributed to the trade by Macmillan

2   4   6   8   10   9   7   5   3   1   paperback

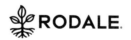

We inspire and enable people to improve their lives and the world around them.

rodalebooks.com

CONTENTS

ACKNOWLEDGMENTS

Just as riding with other, more talented cyclists makes you faster, surrounding yourself with talented, supportive people makes your writing better, too. I've been lucky to have a full pro peloton at my disposal. Leading the way down the road, as always, is my family. Nothing happens without the support of Dave, Juniper, and my mom and dad. On the professional side, thank you to James Herrera, my steady wingman who is always ready with some brilliant programming. Thanks to Shannon Welch and Peter Flax for getting the idea off the ground, and to Natalie Lescroart for shepherding it to the finish line. A tip of my cycling cap to Mitch Mandel, Troy Schnyder, and Christina Gaugler for the lovely design. Thanks also to Mike Yozell and Mike Cushionbury for the tech talk and early reads; to Donna Marlor, Dominique Adair, and Leslie Bonci for the nutritional assistance; and to Hunter Allen and Allen Lim for their cycling training smarts. My deepest appreciation goes to all of you and the many nutritionists, coaches, and researchers who are always willing to pick up the phone and impart their wisdom, and to all the readers and fellow riders who shared their stories. This book is for all of you.

INTRODUCTION
The Need for Speed

Like all good book ideas, the idea for this book came about while I was sipping a double espresso outside a coffee shop on a sunny day. Of course it wasn't just any coffee shop. It was South Mountain Cycles, my hometown bike shop/espresso bar, where fast riders of all shapes and stripes begin and end many a ride.

I was sitting with my editor Shannon Welch, brainstorming ideas for books. It won't surprise you that weight loss came up more than once. Everyone loves a weight loss book. But I've "been there, done that," as they say, and I didn't think I could bring anything fresh to the topic so soon. As we sat in contemplative silence watching the traffic spin by, I focused my stream of consciousness on what cyclists want and talk about most often. A punked-out biker on a crotch rocket roared by. And, just like that, it came to me. When I hear the chatter of riders here and abroad, there's a common theme. Speed.

"Bobby Lea is *flying* right now!"

"That new [fill in hot new bike of the year] is wicked fast."

"Dude, that descent down Dogwood? Scary fast."

"Freakin' Cheryl just sailed up Monster Trail today. How does she do that?"

Cyclists like speed because fast is fun. It's what puts the proverbial wind through our hair and the endorphins in our veins. And the best part: It's something every rider can have. I don't care if you're 30 pounds overweight or 30 years older than you used to be. I don't care if you've been riding for years or just tossed a leg over a bike last Tuesday. You can obtain and enjoy some big-toothy-grin-inducing speed.

In keeping with its Get Fast! goal, this book won't make you wait until you've read the whole thing or followed one of its structured plans to gain speed. No matter who you are or how fast you currently spin those pedals, you can open the book to any page and find a quick tip that will make you faster right now.

LOOKING TO MERCKX (AND BEYOND)

Ask most riders how to get faster and they'll go all Eddy Merckx on you: "Ride lots." That's true. Sort of. But turning up the volume doesn't automatically ramp up your speed. I, and I'm sure you, know many a rider who logs so many miles in the quest for "lots" that they actually start going backward and get slower rather than faster. Maybe you are that rider.

That's because getting fast doesn't stop at putting in miles. In fact, it doesn't even really start there. It starts with your frame. And I don't mean your bike. I see countless riders who can turn their cranks plenty fast, but they can't sustain any real speed because their bodies start shutting them down—mostly in the form of back pain, though cranky hips and achy knees are common speed stealers as well. Your body is like your bike. To go fast it needs to be light, strong, and stable. You wouldn't want to hammer on a cracked frame, right? Well, you can't expect your body to support powerfully churning pistons if you have weak links. Before you can go fast, you need to be strong. The exercises starting on page 60 (many of which pro riders swear by) will get you there.

Likewise, you won't go very fast for very long if your frame is weighed down with the wrong stuff. Cyclists tend to become very fixated on the number on the scale, sometimes to the point of counterproductivity. Though lighter does tend to equal faster, there's a point of diminishing returns where you start sacrificing strength. Remember, cycling performance is determined by a two-sided equation that includes power and weight. To get fast, you need to personalize (and maximize) yours. That's why on page 95 you'll find a simple equation that matches your ideal weight to your cycling goals. This isn't a book about getting skinny; it's one about getting strong and getting fast. Which brings us to fuel.

You already know that, like the gas you put in your car, the fuel you put in your body has a huge impact on your performance. But the gas tank analogy is woefully oversimplified. Whether your four-wheeled machine purrs when you put the pedal down, holds highway speeds without rattling apart, and sails through rough conditions without stalling out on the roadside comes down to more than swinging into a gas station to fill up before a long trip. It's what you've put under the hood, too. Your oil, coolant, lubes, even wiper fluid, can all determine how fast you can drive under different conditions. The same holds true for your body. You have moving parts that need lubricating, spark plugs that need tending, filters that need flushing, and a radiator that needs cooling. It all comes down to what you eat and when you eat it (as well as perhaps a few pills and potions; legal, of course).

Speed also comes down to how you think. In the past few years, exercise scientists have learned that when it comes to sports performance, perception is very much reality—a reality that we often create. For instance, remember last time you bonked? You would have bet your 401(k) that there was nothing but crumbs and vapors left in your muscle stores, right? Most of us have learned what sports researchers call the "limitations theory": that we hit the wall because our muscles have reached their limits and are either out of fuel or screaming uncle from metabolic waste. But none of that is really true.

Even at the end of your hardest century, your glycogen stores aren't tapped out, and there's always more than enough fat to burn. Consider what happens when you learn you have just 1 mile to go in said grueling century. You suddenly find wings and can haul ass to the finish line to the applause of awaiting spectators. That feat would be physically impossible if muscle fatigue were the sole shut-down factor. In short, even when you feel completely done in, there's potential that's untapped.

Finally, getting fast means riding fast. At least as fast as you want, if not faster. So if you want to be a rider who routinely averages 18 mph, you have to occasionally crank it up to 20+. That means tar-geted hard efforts designed to turn up your mphs where you need them most. Are you a slow starter? We can fix that. Do you shoot out like a rocket but fizzle like a cheap sparkler 45 minutes in? We can fix that, too. Different intervals train various physiologic capacities. Shorter, all-out efforts build your total oxygen consumption (VO_2) and explosive power. Longer efforts create muscular endurance. The right blend gives you all the speed you need when you need it most, like bridging gaps, making a break, staying with the leaders on a sustained climb, or sprinting for the line. Even if you never race, that deep reservoir of speed will give you the reserve you need to cruise through your favorite ride in record time.

That's why three chapters of this book are devoted to *you*. It's a soup-to-nuts look at your human machine, what makes it tick, and everything you as a cyclist need to do to make it tick faster for the riding you do. In the spirit of the speed theme, I'll be sure to cut to the chase and give you a shot of science with all the actionable advice you can use. Follow these tips and you'll be flying on the road, dirt, dirt road, 'cross course, track—anywhere and everywhere you love to ride most.

RIDE LIKE YOU'RE FAST (AND YOU'LL BE FAST)

Watch a fast rider in motion and you'll see more than speed. You'll see seamless shifting, braking, cornering, and general bike handling. There's a steadiness and smoothness on the bike that doesn't waste a single watt.

When you consider that an act as subtle as pulling your elbows closer to your body can shave wind resistance enough to increase your speed $\frac{1}{2}$ mile per hour without your working any harder, you can see the potential speed gain from even the most minute adjustment: How and when to jump and dump gears. When it's faster to jam the brakes rather than feather them. How to find the sweet spot in the pack so you can watch your speedometer climb as your heart rate descends. Part 1 of this book is dedicated to detailing all the secrets to fast bike riding and handling so you can pick up a few extra mphs even before you do a single interval.

Once you've learned how to coax every ounce of easy speed from your bike, you'll learn how to make your bike itself faster. This book isn't going to tell you to buy a $10,000 carbon fork, frame, and wheelset, though that is a quick (if not exactly easy) way to get faster. It will tell you how to maintain your current steed so it hums as you hammer. (The difference between a grimy chain and a shiny one can be a few watts . . . Simple solution: Simple Green). I'll also give you industry insights on what upgrades can turn a Cat 5 clunker into a racy semipro.

IT'S NOT JUST ABOUT THE BIKE

Motoring down the road at 25 mph is exhilarating, as is nabbing points in your local criterium series, and finally (finally!) not getting dropped like a safe on the Saturday morning "A" ride. Riding fast is more than fun, however. It's also really good for you (and I mean more than just your ego . . . though, hey, confidence boosting should not be underrated).

Riding hard and fast keeps you healthy and young. In a 20-year study that began with more than 960 men and women ages 50 and older, Stanford University researchers found that the ones who reported doing regular vigorous activity were not only leaner but also had less than half the mortality rate and started experiencing age-related disability a full 16 years later than those who lived in the slow lane.

A Quest for Fast

When I told my husband that I'd signed a contract for a book called *Get Fast!,* he asked if it was a memoir. I laughed, but he had a point. I'd spent the better part of 4 years in the studied pursuit of speed.

It started with a lark. I'd always wanted to do an Ironman and I found this program that promised I could be ready in just 16 weeks. I was a terrible swimmer at the time, so I got a swim coach who connected me with her husband, who was an Ironman coach. He viewed my past race results and thought I had a real shot at qualifying for the Ironman World Championship in Kailua-Kona, Hawaii. Goodbye, 16-week completion program. I set out on an 8-month path that included steps very similar to the ones you'll find here.

First, I decided to get fit. My mission was to make myself strong, quick, and agile—to build a rock-solid foundation that could withstand the weight of all the training bricks I would be laying down on it. That meant thrice-weekly core work, strengthening the supporting cast of muscles from my ankles up, and some explosive plyometrics.

Then I looked at my diet. I've always eaten more like a cornerback than a cheerleader. But the risk of piling my plate like an offensive lineman becomes increasingly high when the training (especially the intensity) ramps up. This is how one ends up actually gaining weight despite burning the equivalent of a double cheeseburger in calories each day. So, using the latest science, I plotted out a food strategy that fueled

Speed makes you healthier right down to the cellular level, an effect that is even more pronounced in the face of stress (and heck, none of us have any of that in our lives, do we?). In a study of chronically stressed workers, researchers from the University of California at San Francisco found that those who blew out their stress with vigorous exercise for 45 minutes 3 days a week had cells that showed fewer signs of aging compared to those who had no physical outlets. Spicing your riding with full-throttle, high-intensity efforts also reduces your risk for heart disease, diabetes, and cancer better than a steady diet of easy riding.

my workouts, aided my recovery, and made me happy without making me huge. (You'll find it and more starting on page 103.)

Finally, I layered on structured intervals—complete with ample amounts of rest and recovery. It worked. I was the second woman and eighth overall finisher in my first priority Olympic distance race, behind a woman who would eventually become a pro triathlete. My time was 23 minutes faster than the previous year. The best part was that I'd clocked a 1:08:52, around 21.7 mph, on the super-hilly 40-K bike course.

As I started to see real results, I wanted to reward all that hard-earned fast with some easy speed. I went ahead and got an aerodynamic helmet, picked up some lighter (though still durable) tires, and got a bike fitting to optimize my position over 112 miles.

Did I get world-class fast? Of course not. But I got really-fast-for-me fast (which, let's face it, is all any of us can ask for). Fast enough to win my age group in Louisville, fast enough to compete in Kona 6 weeks later, and fast enough to enjoy some personal bests in mountain bike races in the years that followed.

Most important, that year I devoted to getting fast taught me lessons I'll have for life. Speed ebbs and flows with the seasons and cycles of life. Racing has its ups and downs. But I will always know the feeling of meeting my potential, of flying as fast as my wheels will take me, and now I understand how to find that place again. My hope and goal is that you will, too.

A nice hard hammerfest is good for your head as well. That euphoria that seeps through you after a spirited ride is your brain playing bartender and serving up an intoxicating cocktail of soothing chemicals such as serotonin, dopamine, and norepinephrine. Just three 45-minute interval sessions a week (like those found starting on page 240) are enough to reduce symptoms of depression as effectively as prescription antidepressants, with far better side effects. As if that weren't enough, vigorous exercise, such as cycling, helps boost levels of growth factors in your brain, which helps create new brain cells and establish new connections between brain cells to boost your cognitive ability.

Ride hard. Get fast. Live longer, better, and smarter. What's not to love?

Note: This book was going into final pass right as the bottom fell out of pro cycling in an unprecedented tidal wave of doping confessions and crackdowns throughout the Pro Tour peloton that was so damaging it resulted in Lance Armstrong being fully stripped of his Tour titles and sponsorships. The original manuscript included a number of references to Lance as well as other pro riders of that era, many of whom I've interviewed and written about over the years. After much consideration, I removed the references where I no longer felt they were appropriate. But I didn't erase every single one.

Yes, there was widespread use of performance-enhancing drugs and blood packing procedures. But that doesn't mean those riders weren't training their brains out, strengthening their core muscles, working on technique, and doing all the hard work required to win Grand Tours. I am in no way defending them or particularly heralding them in the references that remain. But all the EPO in the world doesn't replace 20 to 30 hours a week of structured training, proper diet, and attention to detail. We can still learn from that. We should also take to heart the larger message that while getting fast is fun and rewarding, sacrificing your morals to get there strips it all away. Ride on.

PART 1

FAST TECHNIQUE

Pick up some easy speed—RIGHT NOW!

Your bike wants to go fast.
It's the rider that slows it down.

—Mark Weir, downhill and endurance champion

"You've *got* to take those faster!" barked Ron Ritzler, an otherwise mild-mannered product manager at component manufaturer SRAM, as I once again ground down to banana slug speed through an impossibly tight 180-degree hairpin turn.

"I *would* if you told me *how!*" I returned in my finest pit bull.

And so it went. As I soon discovered, there may be no better place to learn how to get fast than at 6,500 feet in the air—which is precisely where I was (along with Ron) in June 2010, while attending a 3-day training camp that commenced with a run at the Mt. Ashland Super D, a 12-mile, 5,000-vertical-foot plunge down one of Oregon's most demanding racecourses.

Though I have long prided myself on being fairly accomplished in the personal training elements of getting fast, I'll confess to having been less astute at some of the finer points—e.g., technique. Sure, I was good at the basics of shifting, tucking, and drafting. But there are so many technique finesses from the dramatic to the nearly infinitesimal that can deliver easy, immediate speed, sans training, that I could (and did) commit myself to doing better.

Two tips I learned that fateful day in Oregon (where I managed a respectable eighth place in the elite Super D, thank you very much): brake later (and harder) and lead with my "third eye." I was braking well ahead of the hairpin and scrubbing so much speed by the time I got there that the turn wasn't any easier. In fact it was harder because braking too much brings your bike upright and makes negotiating tight turns trickier. I was frustrated. Ron, behind me and forced to slow to an unmanageable speed himself, was frustrated. Finally he delivered some concrete advice: "Carry speed farther into

the turn. Brake hard at the turn. Then let go and lean hard into it."
Now this is the kind of advice that is easy to dish out (and makes
perfect logical sense) but is a little scary to apply. So I waited until I
had a stretch of trail with no one (*ahem*, Ron) close by and that had
some good bailout points if I blew it, and I gave it a whirl.

The braking part worked well, but I was still toppling around like
a daisy in the wind trying to execute the turn. That is until another
speedy descender, local pro Lindsey Voreis, zoomed by and piped up
with further advice: "Use your third eye!" She proceeded to show me
that your third eye is your navel. Your bike will go where your third
eye goes, so you need to point it in the same direction as the two in
your head. This, combined with the braking advice, worked like
magic. I actually began coaching myself out loud during the next
runs: "Third eye! Lean! Third eye!" Come race day, I had the same
fitness I arrived with, but I was measurably faster.

INSTANT GRATIFICATION

Truth be told, I wasn't going to lead with this section of the book. I
was going to be all personal fitness trainer and lead with the advice
you'll find in the second section—Fast Body—which details all the
ways to make your body stronger to get faster. But my husband,
Dave, convinced me otherwise.

"My one little beef," he said, treading very carefully and diplomati-
cally into his critique as he read my first draft, "is you lead with the
stuff that most of us understand we'll need to do but don't want to hear
about right out of the gate—the gym and body work. I want to ride my
bike. I love riding my bike. How can I get faster while riding my bike?"

I resisted saying, "Intervals!" which of course come later, and
thought, "Technique!" I told Dave about the third eye and the payoff
was immediate. He could carry more speed into, through, and out of
corners. He got faster, just like that.

The chapters that follow deliver detailed, expert advice on everything technique related, from shifting and braking to positioning yourself in just the right place in the pack. You'll learn which aerodynamic position produces the biggest power gains (*hint:* it's not what you'd expect) as well as a prerace ritual that can improve your time trial power output by 3 percent.

You can't beat easy speed. Turn the page to get some . . . fast.

1

Fast Riding Tips

How to pedal, shift, and hit the brakes to keep your wheels spinning at top speed.

Fast Fact: The derailleur wasn't allowed in the Tour de France until 1937. (Riders used to have to stop and flip their rear wheel, which had a climbing gear on one side and a downhill gear on the other.) Not surprisingly, the winner's average speed didn't break 20 mph until after that.

How fast you ride isn't really about the bike (though not having to stop and flip a wheel every hill sure does help). It's about *how you ride* the bike you have. I've been left in the dust by madly talented riders piloting trash-picked bikes, and I've watched a grown man in an aero helmet and singlet push a tricked-out $8,000 time trial bike (disc wheel and all) up a hill after all his sloppy shifting and gear grinding finally left him with a broken chain.

How you apply pressure to your pedals, what gears you choose to use, how smoothly you transition from stopping to starting, and how frequently you lay on the brakes all have a huge impact on your final speed. Whether you're a fresh-off-the-bike-shop-floor newbie or a been-around-the-block masters rider, refining your riding style can reward you with easy speed. Here's what you need to know.

PICTURE-PERFECT PEDALING

You've no doubt been told to "pedal circles" a million times. The perfect spin is the holy grail of cycling technique. Everyone agrees that a smooth, evenly powered pedal stroke is not only a thing of beauty but also the pinnacle of efficiency—allowing you to ride faster with less exertion. What they don't always agree on is how to accomplish it.

The ultimate goal is to eliminate as many "dead spots" in the pedal stroke as possible, so at no point are your legs just coming along for the ride, but rather they are always on task propelling you forward.

Years ago, some experts recommended milking every ounce of power through the entire pedal stroke with a technique called ankling. Riders using this technique would actively flex their ankle back and forth during the pedal stroke, so that as their foot came up over the top of the pedal stroke, they'd push down with their heels and lift up with their toes, pulling the pedal down with the weight on their heels. As the pedal came around the bottom, they'd extend their foot, pushing down and around with their toes. It sounds good in theory, but it led to some nasty cases of Achilles tendonitis.

Instead, use those ankles wisely, but less dramatically, to provide a constant power-transferring platform throughout the entire revolution. This modified ankling technique was analyzed by Todd Carver, a biomechanics expert at Retül in Boulder, Colorado. He found that it can help you churn out the same wattage at a heart rate about five beats per minute lower. That means you can maintain the same speed longer. Or turn it up a bit to go faster at the same exertion. To do it:

ALIGN YOURSELF. We don't refer to our pedaling legs as pistons for nothing. From head-on, that's what your legs should look like, straight up and down and with no flapping knees or wobbling hips. Your hip, knee, and ankle should line up throughout the pedal stroke. Park your trainer in front of a mirror sometime and check out your pedaling form. (Note that if you have bowed legs or other unique biomechanical characteristics, you may be an exception here.)

DROP SLIGHTLY AT 12 O'CLOCK. The top of the pedal stroke is where you produce the most power. Maximize it by putting as many muscles as possible into action—including your glutes, hamstrings, and calves—by dropping your heel slightly as you come over the top of the stroke. Your toes will naturally be pointed a little down as you come past 12 o'clock. Dip your heel so your foot is parallel or just a bit below parallel on the downswing.

SCRAPE THE SHOE. As you come through the bottom of the stroke, follow the classic Greg LeMond advice to "act like you're scraping mud off the bottom of your shoe" by engaging your calf muscles to pull through and point your toe down about 10 degrees.

BRING YOUR KNEES TO THE BAR. The upstroke is where everyone loses a little momentum and power because of a tendency to come out of alignment as their knees track laterally (away from the bike). Minimize that by consciously working on an active upstroke. As you begin to come across the top of the stroke, visualize driving your knee forward toward the bar. This helps lighten the pressure on the pedal coming up the back of the pedal stroke, so the one pushing down has less work to do. This also helps to improve hip, knee, and foot alignment, as it stops the knee from tracking laterally (kicking to the outside). The end result is a more efficient pedal stroke with each leg doing less fatiguing work. Be sure to keep your pelvis rock steady in the saddle throughout the whole stroke so there's no wasted energy.

Take It Off Road

Want to develop a silky smooth spin without worrying about mirrors, ankle angles, or foot position? Go mountain biking. Or ride your road bike on some rough dirt roads. Inconsistent terrain demands consistent pedaling effort and forces you to maintain traction and forward momentum without skidding or stalling out. For the best results, find some tricky climbs that will really put your pedaling prowess to the test.

THE "CORRECT" CADENCE

Thanks to Lance, we all were indoctrinated with the 90 rpm gospel. You know the story by now. Lance burst back on the scene postcancer and was spinning the pedals at a lightning-quick cadence of 100 rpm, sometimes higher, while Big Jan Ullrich churned a bigger gear closer to 80 rpm. Lance bested him, so everyone started theorizing that faster was better . . . and faster. Well, not so fast.

Your optimal pedal cadence depends upon myriad factors, including your muscle fiber composition, the type of cycling you're doing, your gear selection, and even your age. Whether you apply very little or a whole lot of force to your pedals determines what muscle fibers you use and what energy stores you draw from to keep going. The same is true for how quickly or slowly you turn your legs around.

When you spin a high cadence (say, 100 rpm and above) in a moderately light gear, you rely mostly on your aerobic, fat-burning energy system to do the work. Low cadences in bigger gears tap into your anaerobic, glycogen-burning system. In a head-to-head study between the two, researchers had riders pedal the same speed for 30 minutes, but one group pushed a light gear at 100 rpm while the other cranked a big plate at 50 rpm. In the end, the two groups displayed nearly identical oxygen-consumption rates as well as very similar heart rates, lactate levels, and power production. What was different between the two groups was energy use. The low-cadence crankers burned through their glycogen stores (particularly in the fast-twitch power fibers) at a much greater rate, while the spinners used mostly fat, sparing their precious glycogen stores. As you deplete your fast-twitch fibers, they become weaker, so your body starts calling in more fibers to do the work, which, as you'd imagine, fatigues you faster. However, it's important to note that high-cadence pedaling tends to be less efficient, and studies show that performance decreases and cardio workload increases as you push into the high-cadence ranges.

That's why most of us find the pedaling sweet spot—where we're neither frying our muscles nor wearing ourselves out—between those two ends of the spectrum. Most coaches recommend about 90 rpm. Researchers have found that cyclists told to choose their most comfortable cadence tend to spin the cranks around 80 rpm (though it's important to note that studies are done on trainers in the lab, which is different than riding a bike down the road; many riders spin more slowly on the trainer because the trainer adds its own layer of resistance). Other research finds that older riders tend to be optimally efficient at lower cadences than their younger counterparts.

In the end, choose a cadence that fits the work you need to accomplish and how you feel. A recent article by Australian researchers, aptly titled "Optimal Cadence Selection During Cycling," sums it up nicely:

➤ *Very high cadence (100 to 120 rpm):* Hammering at this pedal rate can maximize power output and reduce muscle force and neuromuscular fatigue, but it can waste quite a bit of energy, so it's best used for short sprints. (You'll note that track cyclists spin incredibly fast.)

➤ *Moderately high cadence (90 to 100 rpm):* Crits, mountain bike races, cyclocross races, and any longer duration events where you need to spare energy by being more efficient are best served with a brisk cadence, which is less muscle fatiguing.

➤ *Moderate cadence (70 to 90 rpm):* If you're going to be out there for a long time, such as touring or ultraendurance riding, you'll likely benefit from taking your cadence down another notch to the moderate range, which improves economy and lowers energy demands, so you have more reserves for the long haul.

WEAR OUT YOUR GEARS

Ned Overend said it first and it remains true today: Unless you live, ride, and race where the terrain resembles a pancake house breakfast special, you should shift so much that you wear out your gears. Here are some tips for mastering your shifts.

KEEP YOUR CADENCE. Many riders are one-geared wonders. They grind up every rise, loading their legs with lactate, and then jam like a jackhammer on the flats, which sends their heart rate soaring. Both slow you down and wear you out. In general, you should make it your goal to maintain a steady and consistent pedaling cadence. As soon as you feel the pressure on your pedals—change enough for your cadence to slow down or speed up—shift! You'll fatigue much less quickly and maintain a better cruising speed.

LET YOUR LEGS AND LUNGS BE YOUR GUIDE. Remember how high-cadence riding uses your aerobic system, while low-cadence pedaling pulls more power from your muscles? Shift according to how you're feeling to keep going fast with the energy you have. If your thighs are as fried as Kentucky chicken, shift into those small gears to give your legs a rest. Don't have the lungs? Toss it into a larger gear and lower your cadence to bring your heart rate down.

ANTICIPATE THE SHIFT. When I first started racing, I was queen of the suicide shift—I'd wait so long to change gears that my chainrings would be groaning under the stress by the time I'd try some last-second emergency gear change. Inevitably, I'd drop the chain midhill, jam, and go toppling. Fortunately, I got smarter and smoother and now dump one (or more) gears in a split second before powering up a rise or out of a corner.

There are a few key instances where you should always anticipate the shift. For example, before you stand on a climb, shift into a harder gear. Then shift into an easier one when you sit back down. Shift down as you coast to a stop so you can get rolling again without mashing the pedals. Shift when you go into a turn so you can pedal out of it.

CHANGE GEARS. Living, working, and riding near the *Bicycling* magazine offices, as well as one of the country's legendary velodromes, I'm surrounded by gearheads. And I'll confess that I spent a long time letting all of the gear-ratio chatter float over and around me as I nodded and shrugged on cue. Then I did the Mt. Washington Auto Road Bicycle Hillclimb. A couple of weeks before the climb, my husband, Dave, who would also be riding, was diligently preparing his bike, swapping his road setup for a compact crankset, studying the mountain's gradients, and hitting the hills to practice. I felt fit enough, but I hadn't thought twice about my bike. "Do I need a compact?" I asked my friend Bill, who'd done the climb twice. "Nah," he said. "You'll be fine with your thirty-nine." I asked a few others. Everyone said I'd be fine. I decided to leave it be and "run what I brung," so to speak.

I was at peace with that decision until Brian, our friend and chauffeur for the day, Dave, and I pulled up to the venue. I looked at the start, which was easily 12 percent. I looked at Brian. "It's pretty much that way all the way to the top, until it turns to twenty-two percent," he said with a smile. I was out of gears within 30 seconds from the start and spent the day muscling my way up the mountain. I've since paid far more attention to the gear conversations and my own gear conversions, especially when I'll be racing in the mountains.

If you've never switched cassettes, try it sometime. I've seen riders who were way off the back in their 11-23s switch to a 12-27 and suddenly ascend like they had wings. How do you know if your gears are right for you? Ask. What do the other riders in your group run? Do you always seem to be searching for a gear you don't have? Are you completely clueless about gears? It's not as complicated as it seems. For chainrings, the larger the number, the harder it is to pedal and vice versa. For cogs on your cassette, the opposite applies. Larger cogs are easier to pedal than smaller ones. So if you can barely turn over a 23 up the hill, try a 25.

Which leads to the question of whether to run a standard or compact crank. This decision is as ego-driven as any in the cycling world. Many riders still believe that "real cyclists" use standard 53/39 cranksets and that running compact 50/34 cranks implies weakness or newness, neither of which is prized in cycling circles.

The fact is, if you ride where there are plenty of steep pitches and/or you're not a racer who needs a 53/11 to sprint to the finish, a compact may be a wise choice because it allows you to access lower gears to spin up climbs and keep your legs fresh. With the right cassette in the rear, you can really get the best of both worlds. As mentioned above, you can get two, an 11-23 to hammer the flats and a 12-27 to crush the climbs.

HIT THE BRAKES

Braking in and of itself isn't going to make you faster, obviously. But smart braking will, because you're less likely to slow down more than you need and expend more energy than you should getting back up to speed. The right braking will also make you a smoother, more consistent, and—ultimately—safer rider. Here's how to stop better so you can go faster.

LIGHT AS A FEATHER. In most instances (unless you're actually coming to a complete stop for a signal or an intersection), you want to just scrub speed rather than come to a complete halt. That requires a light touch. So light, in fact, that it's called feathering. To feather your brakes, you pull just gently enough so the pads caress the rims. If you feel your weight shift forward, you're pulling too hard.

Feathering takes just one finger to accomplish, maybe two. Keep most of your fingers wrapped around the bar and use just your index finger, or your index and middle finger, to work the brake lever. In this position, you have maximum control of your bike and are less likely to grab a fistful of brakes and stop too abruptly. If you can't reach or it's too difficult to pull the lever with just one or two fingers, ask your bike shop to adjust your levers, or inquire about short-reach levers for smaller hands.

SHIFT BACK. When you hit the brakes, your bike slows down but your body keeps going—sending your weight forward over the front wheel and making it difficult to steer. Counter this effect by shifting your weight back on the saddle as you brake.

USE THE FRONT . . . WISELY. About 70 percent of your braking power comes from the front brake. It's your most powerful ally for scrubbing speed. Don't be afraid to use it; most experienced cyclists primarily use the front brake. The key is to manage your weight distribution while braking. Because you're stopping the front wheel, your body will continue moving forward. Shift your weight back, lower your body (and hence your center of gravity), and use your arms to brace yourself against the deceleration. New riders often don't like to descend on their drops, but it's the safest position for descending. Your weight is back and low, and you have good leverage to pull the brakes and brace your body in the proper position.

A couple of exceptions apply; when it's slippery, for example. Your front brake isn't likely to cause a skid on dry surfaces. It can most definitely cause a skid on slippery ones, though, and a front wheel skid almost inevitably leads to a fall. Also, bumpy descents require judicious use of the front brake. Your wheels can bounce off the pavement during these descents. You want them to be able to keep rolling when they make contact again. And momentum is your best friend over rough terrain because it keeps you upright and moving forward. Hitting the front brake kills momentum and makes it harder to control the bike.

When heading into a turn, use the front and rear brakes more evenly as you scrub speed to reduce the likelihood of either wheel skidding. You can brake very lightly in a turn, but it's best to lay off the brakes entirely and let the bike roll.

WORK THEM MORE WHEN WET. It takes longer to stop on wet roads. The roads are slick and your rims are less grippy, so they won't work as well. When tackling a long descent or twisty road in the wet, keep your brakes ever so slightly squeezed. This helps keep them free from excess water and allows for quicker stopping. Also, keep your bike more upright when braking to prevent skidding out.

PULL THE E-BRAKE. Sometimes you've got to slam on the brakes, like when a car door swings open directly in your path. To pull an emergency stop, place both feet parallel to the ground, lift your butt, and shift your weight way back behind the saddle. Extend your arms and sink your weight low, dropping your torso toward the top tube; then give your brakes a tight squeeze. Do this all in one smooth move, so it almost looks like you're trying to throw your bike forward, and hurl your body back. It's fun to practice in parking lots, and you never know when you might need it. It makes you faster by saving you time picking yourself off the pavement.

2

Up and Over

Tackle mountains (up, around, and down) with these fast climbing, cornering, and descending tips.

Fast Fact: Increasing your power just 5 percent on the climbs and conserving just 5 percent on the descents can make you nearly a minute and a half faster over the course of a hilly 10-K ride.

—Paraphrased from D. P. Swain, "A Model for Optimizing Cycling Performance by Varying Power on Hills and in Wind" in *Medicine and Science in Sports and Exercise*

There's a saying that races are won and lost in the mountains (the Tour de France comes to mind). Most people assume that's because the climbing specialist can simply leave the other riders crawling against the anchors of gravity. That's true . . . sometimes. But if ascending "like a homesick angel," as cycling broadcasters would say, is all it took to cross the line first, whippet-thin pedalers like the Schleck brothers would win every time. Instead, racers like Cadel

Evans, who are skilled bike handlers as well as climbers, are the ones who steal the show.

This is a lesson I've learned, and continue to learn, the hard way (and it's especially true on a mountain bike, where technical terrain comes into play). The starkest example was the BC Bike Race, a mountain bike stage race in British Columbia that is riddled with long, often hairy descents down the Canadian mountain ranges. Stage after stage, I found myself sailing up the hills past scores of fellow racers only to find myself feeling like just another obstacle on the trail as they came screaming past on the descents.

I've since worked on my descending and cornering (both on and off road), and my improved ability has meant the difference between holding on to a podium position or ultimately being tossed off the back. I'm also far less sore and spent after a long day in the saddle. When you can relax, stay loose, roll through corners, and sail down mountainsides, you have far more energy to burn at the end of the day, which makes it easier to hang with (and maybe even beat) some of your faster buddies. Here's some expert advice for getting up, over, and down the mountains faster.

RULE THE CLIMBS

You already know that much of your speed on ascents depends on the numbers on the scale. It is true that the ruling force of gravity creates a caste system in our sport, designating some of us slaves to its downward pull while others fly unfettered to be kings and queens of the mountains. Fortunately, cycling is not a feudal (or futile) sport, and there are myriad tips and techniques that will help you ascend the ranks no matter what you weigh. Here's how to flatten even the steepest hills to get to the top faster.

FLOAT LIKE A BUTTERFLY. You can't change your weight on a climb, but you *can* change how heavy you ride. Instead of death-gripping the handlebar, clenching your teeth, and mashing your way up the mountainside, practice what Andy Applegate, an elite-level coach who teaches climbing skills in Asheville, North Carolina, calls "qigong climbing." It is a moving meditation that enhances mind-body connection and promotes relaxation, thus giving your body more energy for the task at hand. It works like this:

➤ As you approach the climb, think "light" thoughts. Picture butterflies, birds, clouds, and being weightless in the wide-open sky. Likewise, keep those thoughts positive. If you're thinking, "I'm going to get my butt handed to me again," you likely will. If you think, "I can do this climb," you will as well. Sounds corny, but try it. It works.

➤ Position yourself for maximum oxygen consumption. Keep your back straight and chest open. Relax your arms so your elbows are outside of your hips.

➤ Starting at the top of your head, progressively relax your body. Relax your forehead, eyes, cheeks, mouth, jaws, neck, shoulders, chest, back, arms, and hands. The goal is for your upper body to be so quiet that if someone were to see you from the waist up, they wouldn't know whether you were climbing Mt. Washington or cruising to the coffee shop (this could be a little difficult on parts of Mt. Washington, I'll admit).

➤ Press lightly on the pedals and keep your legs moving rhythmically. Erase every ounce of unnecessary tension.

Some of this may sound new agey, but try it. You'll be surprised how much energy you have to climb even the hardest hill when you're not wasting energy with negative thoughts and tension in your body.

SIT AND SPIN. You'll see pro climbing specialists out of the saddle so much in the mountains it looks like they're running, rather than riding, up them. For most of us mere mortals, however, staying seated and spinning a relatively easy gear (the key word here being *relatively;* see more on that in the next tip) is the better strategy. When you stand, you put more weight on your leg muscles, so they have to work harder, which uses about 10 percent more energy and sends your heart rate about 5 to 10 percent higher. For gradual grades, sit rearward on the saddle. Shift up toward the nose when the going gets steep and gently pull the bars to assist you up the hill.

FLY IN THE FACE OF CW. The idea behind climbing with a small gear and high cadence is that you're tapping into your slow-twitch fibers and aerobic energy system, which have far more reserves than your fast-twitch fibers and anaerobic energy system. But I've never been convinced that it's always beneficial to spin like a hamster in a wheel, especially if your natural inclination (and likely muscle fiber composition) is to push a bigger gear a little slower. A conversation I had with triathlete Chrissie Wellington (who jams a monster gear) confirmed that suspicion. During an interview, she put it like this: "It's a misconception that you need to spin a smaller gear at a higher cadence on the bike. You don't. Doing that actually raises your heart rate and makes you more tired, which doesn't serve you very well in long-distance racing. Cranking it down and pushing a bigger gear lets me lower my heart rate. It's what feels natural to me and enables me to go the fastest I can go." Sounds reasonable to me, and it is advice I personally agree with despite being told to quicken my cadence over the years. My take: Try both and see where you find your sweet spot. In general, you likely want to keep that cadence at or above 70 rpm, even if you go with a bigger gear.

SHIFT BEFORE YOU STAND. Though sitting is more energy efficient, there will be times when getting out of the saddle is in order—like when your body needs a break on a long climb and the pitch becomes so steep you need to recruit every pound to push those pedals, or just when you want to accelerate. To maintain momentum, shift into the next hardest gear before you stand.

Standing in the same gear you're pushing from the saddle will just slow you down and suck your energy. Shift up a gear and stand as your power foot comes to the top of the pedal stroke. This will push you forward and boost your momentum. Stand with your butt right over the saddle and your weight centered over the bottom bracket to keep even traction on the tires. Like a Tour pro climbing Mont Ventoux, you should feel like you're running (or at least jogging) on the pedals. Gently push on the handlebar and rock the bike beneath you as you climb.

HOVER BELOW THRESHOLD. To crest a climb as quickly as you can without blowing up before you hit the top, climb at an intensity that is just below your lactate threshold (where your legs start to burn). Find your ideal climbing intensity by riding a hill as hard as your legs will allow for about 30 to 60 seconds; then back down about 10 percent. That's where you want to be. Hovering here gives you the reserve to dig deep and handle temporary changes in pace or pitch without immediately popping. If you're already at threshold, you have nowhere to go but down.

FLATTEN YOUR FEET. Your feet are the platform putting power into your pedals. The ankles hold them steady while transferring power from the calves. Cycling instructor Tim Pelot, a certified strength and conditioning specialist in Burnsville, Minnesota, once told me he saw a surprising number of riders who lose speed at this key junction. "Those big mashers who pedal with their toes pointing down lose power through their calves," he explained. "Push through the heels or the middle of the feet with your ankles locked to transfer maximum power. By changing feet position, you can find strength you didn't know you had."

SET GOALS. A few of these tips will deliver small instant speed increases. Measurable gains will take a bit more time and practice. Work on hills once or twice a week and set some goals to accelerate your success. "I like very specific goals, like 'I want to climb this hill in my twenty-eight at seventy-five rpm,'" said Pelot. "Those goals help you concentrate on the very things that will help make you a better climber, as opposed to just saying, 'I want to get to the top faster.'" (You'll find specific climbing drills on page 253.)

STRENGTHEN YOUR SUPPORTING CAST. You may have legs of steel, but if your back is as weak as a tin can, you'll stall out on the steep stuff. That's because your back and ab muscles keep your pelvis stable as you pedal. When they start to fatigue, your form deteriorates, your hips rock, and your pain sensors light up. Check out the "The Get Fast! Cycling Core Plan" workout starting on page 60 to keep your support system strong.

WORK THE CLIMB. All climbs are not created equal. Nor should your technique be identical on every grade. Here are a few specific tips to pick up speed on every pitch.

Long, steady climbs: Stay planted in the saddle as long as you are comfortable. Spin a comfortable gear. If the hill is very long, stretch occasionally to prevent tightening up through the torso. Stand and push your hips forward to relieve your lower back. Slide back on the saddle and round your back to stretch the upper back, shoulders, and neck.

Rollers: Momentum is your friend here, which is why even bigger riders can rock the rollers as well as, if not better than, the climbing specialists. Throw the hammer down at the bottom of the roller, gradually increasing your effort as you head upward (it's okay to go a little into the red, since the ascent is short and you have ample recovery on the downside). Stay in the gear you start with and stay seated until your cadence drops. Then stand to keep your cadence. If it drops again, shift. When you can see over the crest, click up a gear and power over the top to pick up momentum to carry you over the other side.

Short and steep: Lower your cadence so as not to spin out and lose momentum. If you're standing, keep your body crouched, with hands on hoods for even weight distribution. While seated, place your hands on the bar top and push your weight back on the saddle for maximum pedaling leverage. Gently pull your elbows in to stiffen your core and deliver more power to your pedals through your legs. If the hill is longer, alternate between sitting and standing to keep your effort consistent. Be sure to lighten up on the pedals a touch before making any shifts to keep the chain from dropping (or worse, snapping).

CARVE THE CORNERS

The road is rarely linear, but rather it is filled with glorious curves. Some are gentle and sweeping like a bunny slope. Others are steep, sharp, and treacherous like a triple black diamond. The skiing analogy is also apt in the risk department. Carrying speed through corners adds up to many seconds, if not minutes, shaved by the end of a long ride or race. Overcooking a turn, however, slows you down in a hurry, as you hit the pavement (or worse). So, needless to say, I'm a big fan of practicing only in the safest places possible, such as a grassy slope or a wide-open swath of pavement that has ample safe bailout sections should you blow it.

Whatever you do, always ride within your comfort level and don't take foolish chances. I have a couple of close friends who have earned ambulance rides after taking turns hotter than they could handle. Unless someone is writing you checks to ride, take your time and let your skills come up to speed at your own comfort level. Here's how to start sweeping through turns with greater ease . . . and speed.

DROP ONTO THE DROPS. You want to keep your center of gravity low and your hands in close contact with the brakes when heading toward a turn. The best place for both is on the drops.

STAY LOOSE. You corner with your whole body—hips, feet, hands, torso. If you tense up and get rigid, you'll end up straightening your arms and pushing the bike to the outside. At best, you'll be fighting your bike through the turn. At worst, you're going down. As you approach a turn, consciously relax your hands and arms so you have a firm (but not tight) grip on the bars and your upper body feels loose.

SCRUB SPEED EARLY. Feather the brakes as you approach the corner, squeezing the levers just enough to caress the rims. You should barely feel your weight going onto your handlebar. If your weight shifts forward, you're squeezing too hard. Braking makes your bike sit up and straighten out—neither will help you negotiate a turn. The goal is to brake enough before the turn so that you can lean and coast through it with minimal (if any) braking before pedaling out of the turn.

Note: Here's where mountain biking rules are a bit different because of the tires and terrain. When you're on the dirt, you can carry your speed longer. Accordingly, brake later (and harder) and whip your bike through the turn with your hips and torso, allowing the back wheel to drift a little. That's possible but considerably more difficult to achieve on skinny tires.

TAKE A WIDE LINE. The fastest way from here to there is a straight line, right? Aim to create one in every turn. Enter the corner as wide as possible (without crossing yellow lines). This reduces the tightness of the curve, so it's less scary. Once in the turn, cut the corner on the inside and exit wide (again without crossing the yellow lines). This will take you in the straightest possible line through the turn.

LEAN THE BIKE, NOT (ALWAYS) YOUR BODY. I'll confess, this one took me a while to get. For gentle turns, it's fine to lean both body and bike. But as they get tighter, you need to keep your body more upright as you lean the machine beneath you (this is also called countersteering). I didn't grasp this out of the gate; hence my first attempts at cornering hard at speed were pretty sketchy as I attempted to make like the motorcycle racers I'd seen tipping so far they skimmed their knee pads on the ground (though I was nowhere near that cool). The results were a bit hairy as my tires broke traction and I had to do some radical braking, shifting, and praying to bring the bike back under me without sailing off the road. I soon learned that while you do want to lean the bike, sometimes sharply, you want to keep your body weight over the centerline of the bike so you keep the tires firmly pressed into the road.

Countersteering is done through a simultaneous series of moves that tilt the bike while keeping your body more upright to maintain traction. Coming into the turn, shift your weight back so it's low over the top tube. Extend your outside leg, pushing very heavily on that pedal as you lightly press down on the handlebar with your inside hand. Drop the other knee to the inside toward your frame, which will automatically shift your hips and shoulders, and thus the bike, into the turn and the direction you want to go.

LOOK AT YOUR EXIT—WITH ALL THREE EYES. Your bike follows your eyes. Look as far through the corner as you can, aiming for a wide arc, so your bike takes the straightest line possible through the curve. Pay attention to what some pros also call your "third eye": your navel. Though it can't really see, it does take you where you want to go when it's "looking" in the right direction.

You ultimately steer your bike with your hips. So by turning your body to bring your third eye in the direction you want to travel, your hips turn with your bike.

PEDAL OUT OF IT. Shift down before you hit the turn. As you exit the curve, start pedaling again to set yourself back up and bring yourself back to speed. For tight corners, which soak up a lot of speed, stand and sprint out of the corner to regain your momentum. This has a side benefit of stretching your back and legs and giving your knees a little relief.

DRILL THOSE SKILLS. Some coaches, like Carl Cantrell of Alamogordo, New Mexico, ask their racers to practice cornering drills, much like swimmers practice their pull and kick and runners do strides. The idea is to make the right motions automatic, so there will be no thinking required when you approach the real thing. Here's what he recommends.

Circles: Put your bike in a low gear and ride in slow left-hand circles, gradually picking up speed and bringing the circle tighter and tighter until you feel the rear wheel break traction. That's your tipping point. Get a feel for that point and get comfortable riding within it. Practice in both directions.

Figure eights: Once you've got circles down, move on to figure eights, which are perfect practice for real-life riding because you have to change directions quickly to maintain control. This is where you should really feel countersteering at work.

DESCEND WITH DEMON SPEED

Okay, *demon speed* may be a little bit of hyperbole. But let's face it, we'd all *like* to rip down the mountain, hair afire. But it can be scary, and as with cornering (especially downhill cornering), you have to carefully weigh the risk with the reward. Learning bike handling skills that make you more comfortable and confident—hence faster—on descents is worthwhile. Throwing caution to the wind? Bad idea.

The most important point here is that the very things nervous descenders do because they're scared are the actions that can cause them to have to fight the bike to the point of fatigue or even loss of control. Such was the case with Kelly, a woman I met on a charity ride in 2011. She was so scared of picking up too much speed on descents that she sat bolt upright and rode her brakes until she smelled rubber. She described her first long mountainside descent as "just awful." "My shoulders were so tensed up, I felt like my traps attached to my ears. I was wearing gloves, but my hands were still completely cramped up and beet red by the time I got to the bottom."

Like climbing and cornering, safe, speedy descending is a matter of weight distribution and control. The easiest place to practice is on a short, relatively straight descent, where you have good sight lines and can aim for the bottom without hitting the brakes. These tips will help.

USE THE BIG RING. A little tension on the chain helps you control the bike. You also might want/need to pedal on the way down to maintain momentum. Either way, it's to your advantage to use a high gear when heading downhill.

HIT THE DROPS. Some riders get nervous about descending on the drops because you pick up speed fast in this very aerodynamic position. But it's a far safer position for descending than on top of the bar. Your hands have much better leverage on the brakes, so you can stop more quickly, and your weight distribution—butt, back, and lower center of gravity—is more stable there than when you are sitting poker straight, when your center of gravity is too high and your weight is often too far forward. (Think which position is more likely to tip forward over the bar . . .)

PUT YOUR BUTT BACK. Shift your rear back on the saddle. This evenly distributes your weight on the back, lowers your center of gravity, keeps the rear wheel firmly on the ground, and makes the bike more predictable and stable. For even more stability, tuck your knees in toward the top tube. This also makes you more aerodynamic.

MAINTAIN A SOLID BUT FLUID PLATFORM. Your feet should be at the three and nine o'clock positions, respectively (unless cornering), so they're parallel to the ground and distributing your weight evenly. Your arms and legs should be firm, but relaxed enough to absorb bumps and road chatter, allowing the bike room to move.

CARESS THOSE RIMS. You don't need a degree in physics to know that jamming on the brakes is a bad idea when you're carrying speed downhill on two wheels. Skidding, endoing (going backend over handlebar), and fishtailing are all unfortunate by-products. Instead, scrub your speed gently (as you would cornering) by feathering the brakes on and off. Remember, your front brake is your friend; just use a light touch. If you find yourself needing to hit your brakes hard, be sure to push your weight back hard to keep your rear wheel down.

PULL YOUR PARACHUTE. This is one of my favorite ways to scrub speed if I find myself going too scary fast. Just think of your body as a parachute and sit taller and wider (putting your elbows out) to catch all the wind you can. You can even stand up on the pedals (but keep your weight back) to increase the resistance. It's an easy way to slow down without braking.

PEDAL...SOMETIMES. There's nothing sweeter than coasting down a long descent, but you don't want to go completely on idle or you'll have to work harder than necessary to get back up to speed. You can use your odometer as a guide. Any time your speed falls below 20 to 25 mph, put your pedals in motion. Anything above that, conserve your energy and coast.

3

Aero Speed

Cheat the wind for easy speed.

Fast Fact: "Over a flat road on a windless day, 90 percent of the resistance impeding forward motion on a bicycle is due to aerodynamic drag."

—Allen Lim, PhD, "Power Basics"

Think for a second about the time and effort you invest in training to get just that little bit faster. You have to sweat out an entire off-season to add 30 watts to your average power output. Now consider this: Lowering your riding position from the hoods to the drops can save 30 to 50 watts at 25 mph, thus saving you 3 to 5 minutes in a 40-K time trial.

That's the power of aerodynamics—as pointed out to me a few years ago (in PowerPoint clarity) by Allen Lim, PhD, training guru to the pros. Maximizing the ease with which you slip through the air becomes even more important as you approach your fitness ceiling, because the gains you'll make through training will become incrementally smaller (though I should note that most of us day-job-holding types aren't exactly bumping into our fitness ceilings with any frequency). As Lim put it, "The gains you make by training someone physiologically are relatively small when you consider that you can make ten, twenty, even thirty percent gains through aerodynamics."

SLICE THROUGH THE AIR

Aerodynamics is the ticket to easy speed. But this is not going to be a chapter instructing you to run out and buy a pointy helmet with a face shield or to spray-glue your race numbers flat on your kits (though those things will make you faster, as will a nice $3,000 disc wheel). What most riders fail to realize as they're forking over their credit cards for tri-spoke wheels is that, all things being equal, your bike is only responsible for about 25 to 30 percent of the speed-slowing aerodynamic drag. Your body accounts for the other 70 to 75 percent. Consider these stats from aerodynamics gurus Jim Martin, John Cobb, and Asker Jeukendrup.

Over a 40-K course, the following aerodynamic swaps can produce these time savings:

➤ Aerodynamic (blade-style) fork vs. round fork: $\frac{1}{2}$ minute

➤ Rear disc and tri-spoke wheels vs. traditional spoke wheels: 1 to $1\frac{1}{2}$ minutes

➤ Aerodynamic (time trial or tri) frame vs. standard road frame: 1 to $2\frac{1}{2}$ minutes

➤ Aero (time trial) bars vs. upright bar: 5 minutes

➤ Aerodynamic tuck position vs. upright riding position: 6+ minutes

Aerodynamic parts most definitely buy you some easy speed, especially in time trials (TT) or triathlons (when you don't have the benefit of a pack to protect you from the wind). But it's your body far more than your bike that's slowing you down. Do the math. You can shave more than twice as much time over a 40-K TT simply by getting into a tuck than you can by buying a pimped-out TT bike with all the wind-cheating bells and whistles.

DUCK AND COVER

As anyone who's ever sat up to slow down knows, your surface area (especially from the front) creates a great deal of resistance against the air. That's why there's such a significant increase in speed when you go from the hoods to the drops. The problem is, there's a diminishing point of speed production as your hip angle decreases and you become too cramped or uncomfortable to breathe deeply and pedal powerfully.

I saw this firsthand during a trip to the A2 Wind Tunnel, a state-of-the-art aerodynamics testing facility in Charlotte, North Carolina, formerly run by Mike Giraud—the same aero guru who has helped dial in numerous pros and the Timex and Saturn racing teams. I was training for an Ironman-length triathlon at the time, so we were trying to find the sweet spot where I was low enough to minimize my wind resistance but not so scrunched up that I couldn't maintain the tuck for 112 miles.

Interestingly, dropping from a fairly upright position to as low as I could go (which I should preface isn't all that low; my hamstrings are flexible, but my back just doesn't round out into a turtle shell position) made a nearly negligible impact on my "aero watts," the number of watts saved through aerodynamics, because my upper body was interfering with my lower body. As my torso dropped, so did my watts. (Of course, while some riders can get very low while still having enough comfortable breathing and pedaling space, others cannot. The sweet spot varies.) What resulted in the most measurable savings of the day was pulling my elbows in as narrow as comfortably possible. Start to finish, the entire wind tunnel adjustment saved 28 aero watts, enough to make me go $\frac{1}{2}$ mph faster without pedaling any harder.

It's also important to realize that the resistance from the air hitting you head-on is only one way air slows you down. An average-sized rider churning along at 20 mph has to displace more than 1,000 pounds of air per minute. That wake creates a big drag on your efforts. That's why time trialists wear skinsuits (tight suits with no pockets in the back to catch the wind), shoe covers, and wraparound glasses to create a clean sweep of air around their bodies with nothing to catch the wind and create more turbulence and drag.

The faster you go, the more drag increases, which is why it becomes exponentially harder to go faster the faster you ride. In turn, that means the faster you ride, the more important good aerodynamics becomes.

HOW LOW CAN YOU GO?

As you'll see in Chapter 5, increasing your range of motion, especially through your hips, glutes, and hamstrings, will allow you to drop closer to your bar while still keeping your pelvis planted squarely on the saddle (which is critical for maintaining full, comfortable pedaling power). You also need strong core muscles to comfortably hold you in that position.

In Part 2, you'll find specific workouts for improving your foundation, core strength, and flexibility. Improving those fitness components will unleash speed you otherwise couldn't sustain. You should also investigate your bike fit. Riders often raise their bars (especially on TT bikes or bikes equipped with aero bars) to open their hip angle. That's one way to accomplish it—though probably not the most aerodynamic approach. Another technique to consider is to ride shorter cranks, which lowers the position of your leg at the top of the pedal stroke, increasing your hip angle by 2 to 3 degrees without raising your bar and torso. TT riders and triathletes will also use this technique when they can't comfortably drop their aero bars any further. By switching their cranks with a pair that's 1 centimeter shorter, they often find they can drop their bars another 1 to 2 centimeters.

As mentioned earlier, for many riders (myself included), making the body position narrower (e.g., pulling in the elbows), not just lower, yields the biggest aero watt gains. On the road, that means being conscious of pulling your elbows in close to your body as you ride rather than letting them chicken wing out into the wind. For time trials and triathlons, it means aero bars.

Though it's true that aero bars can reduce your cycling efficiency, the aerodynamic savings more than make up for it. In one study, cyclists tested on both standard and aero bars lost about 9 watts in efficiency on the aero bars, but they saved 100 watts because of the dramatically reduced drag. Generally speaking, you can expect to drop your 40-K time by about a minute in switching to aero bars. If you don't want to spring for new aero bars for the occasional time trial, opt for a pair of mini clip-ons that attach to your existing bar.

CATCH A DRAFT

The peloton nearly always swallows up the lone fliers for a reason—they're using a fraction of the energy. By riding closely behind another rider, you can use more than 30 to 40 percent less energy as the guy pulling you along—a huge, huge savings. And here's another cool pack-riding fact: Even though it looks like the lead rider is doing all the work, he or she actually benefits from the tagalongs. When a rider pedals closely behind you, he or she reduces the turbulence coming off your back and reduces your drag, so you use about 3 percent less energy than if you were out on a solo cruise.

Unless you're a lone wolf, you've undoubtedly ridden with others and experienced the energy-saving wonders of drafting. But I'll bet that you've also experienced the frustrations of following wheels in a pack. Fact is, while most of us ride pacelines often, unless they're with the same like-minded, familiar riders, they can be tough to follow as they break apart, scrunch up, and generally come undone. Here are a few tips for keeping it together.

KEEP YOUR EYES DOWN THE ROAD. Behave as you would driving in heavy traffic. Don't stare directly at the rider in front of you. Instead, look through the rider in front of you. That way you can look about 10 meters up the road and see the other riders and anticipate what the group will do. This allows you (and everyone else who should be doing this) to ride proactively instead of reactively, which keeps the line moving smoothly.

KEEP THE PACE. It's called a paceline for a reason, yet the number one gaffe riders make is jacking up the speed when they hit the front, sending riders sailing off the back. Sometimes it's an intentional show-off maneuver, but often it's an innocent mistake. Remember, when you're sitting in the line, you're moving at a good clip (let's say 18 to 20 mph) while using 30 to 40 percent less energy than the rider driving the train. The natural instinct when you become the engine is to crank up your effort so as not to slow the train down. Resist. Increase your effort just enough to compensate for the wind and keep it steady. As you're riding through the line, pay attention to the average speed and effort of the group. When you get to the front, maintain that effort.

MICROADJUST. It's practically impossible for everyone to put forth equal amounts of effort, especially on undulating terrain. You need to make microadjustments along the way to prevent the accordion effect—where the line alternately bunches together and then gets strung out with big gaps. Again, it's like driving a car. You don't slam on the brakes, then hit the gas. You modulate your speed. Make minute adjustments in how hard you're pressing down on the pedals, soft-pedaling as necessary. Feather your brakes while you pedal. Sit up and stick your head out in the wind a bit. All these will help keep the effort and pace consistent without causing a yo-yo effect in the line.

HUG THE LINE. As you pull off the front, decelerate just a bit and stay close to the line. You'll still be able to catch a draft as they pedal by, and it will be easier to seamlessly slip in at the back rather than miss the line and have to accelerate to catch back on.

RELAX! You need to be able to hold your line whether it's in a paceline or a group. You can't do that if you're white-knuckling the bars. Holding on too tightly not only wastes energy and ultimately slows you down but also makes you a twitchy rider, since your bike will overreact to your every little movement as you get a drink and look over your shoulder. Your hands should be relaxed enough for you to wiggle your fingers.

FLOW WITH THE WIND. A paceline is perfect for a headwind. But constant crosswinds call for other formations, such as an echelon, which looks like a diagonal slash. So if the wind is coming from the left, the front rider shifts left and the other riders move up, often overlapping the rear wheel of the rider in front of them. Riders take turns pulling off into the direction of the wind. This is effective for aerodynamics, but it is often unrealistic to maintain for long stretches on an open-road group ride. It takes up a huge chunk (if not all) of the lane, which motorists (and traffic laws) generally frown upon. Overlapped wheels are also inherently dangerous since one swerve to miss a pothole can send the whole formation tumbling down. Finally, wind directions can change suddenly as the road turns, rendering the echelon inefficient with a simple turn around a bend. Reserve this formation for long, open straightaways.

PICK YOUR PLACE IN THE PACK. When there are too many riders for an orderly paceline (or in many race situations), you'll find yourself in a pack. The same general rules apply about holding your line and watching your front wheel. You'll also need to pick your place in the pack.

I have to laugh every July as I listen to color commentators announce the Tour de France. After every crash it's the same: "See, that's why you have to ride at the front." As if it's physically possible for every rider to be up there. But to be fair, the front of the bunch (if not actually the front line) is the fastest, most energy-efficient place to be, especially as the road twists and undulates. A pack will go progressively slower through a corner and progressively faster out of a corner, which will leave you feeling completely spent as you alternately slow down and speed up over and over again. The sweet spot in a big pack is in the first 10 to 20 riders. But note, if you're among the first 10 or so, you'll be expected to do your share of the work, taking pulls and closing gaps. If you're not up for that, drift into the 15 to 20 range, where you can sit in.

With experience, you also can use the pack dynamics (and aerodynamics) to your advantage. One way to stay comfortably within the bunch without getting dropped is to learn how to alternately move up and backslide. For example, if there's a hill coming up and you're not the strongest climber, you can move up toward the front in anticipation of the climb, then naturally drop back through the group as the climb wears on (hopefully still having a few wheels to hang on to by the time you crest the climb).

To move to the front, you can move up through the natural gaps that occur in the pack (always looking over your shoulder, of course, to be sure not to cut people off). Or, more simply, move toward the edge of the group and use that as your passing lane. With luck, other riders will be doing the same and you can catch a ride to the front.

4

10 Get Fast! Tricks

Little things can add up to major speed.

> **Fast Fact:** Listening to music increases your muscle force and velocity during explosive workouts. It also helps you clear lactate more quickly during your cooldown (because it keeps you moving).

Sometimes you find untapped speed in the most unexpected places, like in a snug new pair of stiff-soled cycling shoes or in a perfectly executed playlist. The following are 10 places to pick up some easy speed. Some take a little time. Others are as quick and easy as lubing your chain. Here they are in no particular order.

MOVE YOUR CLEATS

Cycling is full of golden rules that riders used to follow without a second thought. Cleat position is one of those. Many riders give their cleat position perfunctory treatment, automatically cinching them down smack-dab in the center of the ball of the foot as they've always been told. That conventional wisdom has been called into question during recent years, as high-profile cycling experts such as Joe Friel, author of the Training Bible series; Götz Heine, former pro cyclist and shoe designer; and Steve Hogg, a world-renowned expert on bike fitting have discovered you can tap into unmined power by simply shifting your cleat position back.

Maybe the most extreme example is Friel himself, who, following a recommendation by Heine, pushed his cleats all the way back to his arch (he blogged about actually punching holes in the soles of his Shimano shoes to do so). The result: He improved his ratio of power to heart rate (a measure of how many watts you're producing relative to how hard you're working) by an impressive 9 percent.

When I asked Hogg about it, he agreed it was an extreme example, but was quick to note that most riders can make performance improvements with a change in cleat position. "I have one elite customer who, after major changes in cleat position, improved his personal best over a forty-three-K TT by three minutes."

Here's how Hogg recommends dialing in your cleats to pick up a little easy speed.

ADJUST THE FORE AND AFT TO FIT YOUR RIDING. Your calf muscles work hard stabilizing your foot on the pedal during cycling. Cleat position fore and aft affects just how hard. The further forward the cleats, the harder the calves need to work. Having them forward does, however, allow you to apply higher peak torque to your pedals. The key is finding the position that will provide the torque you need without the calf fatigue you don't. "I've found over many years and thousands of customers that the great majority of riders perform better with the ball of the foot in front of the pedal axle on a conventional shoe," says Hogg, who recommends the following placement as a starting point.

➤ *Shoe sizes 36–38:* center of ball of foot 7–9 mm in front of the center of the pedal axle

➤ *Shoe sizes 39–41:* 8–10 mm in front

➤ *Shoe sizes 42–43:* 9–11 mm in front

➤ *Shoe sizes 44–45:* 10–12 mm in front

➤ *Shoe sizes 46–47:* 11–14 mm front

➤ *Shoe sizes 48–50:* 12–16 mm in front

Depending on what kind of riding you do, adjust your cleats as follows.

Pure sprinter (e.g., track): Move the cleats forward from the recommendations above. Endurance isn't a major factor in sprinting, so calf fatigue isn't an issue.

Road racer (e.g., crits, day races): Move cleats so that the pedal axle is a bit behind the ball of the foot (as recommended in the chart) to relieve the calves. Rearward cleats will allow your big muscles to work optimally, keep your calves fresher, and still provide plenty of torque for breakaways and finishing sprints.

Time trial rider, distance rider, 24-hour mountain bike racer: If you need to ride hard and/or long and have little need for sudden acceleration, move your cleats even farther back toward the mid-foot. Some riders find this position also helps them eliminate "hot foot" and other painful foot conditions that arise from pressure on the feet.

Remember, if you move the cleats back any meaningful amount, you will need to drop your saddle accordingly.

PRECOOL YOUR JETS

When I was doing triathlons, I always noticed how good—really good—I felt on the bike fresh out of a nice cool body of water. I felt like I could go faster longer even on the hottest July days without melting (and slowing) down. So I started mimicking that experience whenever I could, most notably soaking myself in the pool each morning before lining up for the Trans-Sylvania Mountain Bike Epic, where I'd be racing my mountain bike for four hours in 85 suffocatingly humid degrees.

You'll see plenty of pros employing the same, albeit more high-tech, strategy. Adam Craig was photographed wearing an ice vest at the start of the blisteringly hot 2011 Mellow Johnny's Classic pro cross-country race in Johnson City, Texas. The US triathlon team used the same vests to precool their cores during the 2004 Olympics in steamy Athens. Trainer Allen Lim, PhD, also has riders cool their cores during competition by drinking plenty of cold fluids and dumping water over their heads, necks, and backs. Of course this isn't rocket science. But there is some impressive science about how you can use said cooling strategies to get faster when it's hot.

In a study of 12 trained cyclists, researchers set the lab temperatures at about 90 degrees with 55 percent humidity and had the riders perform a 46.4-kilometer simulated time trial course that included two climbs. The researchers brought the riders back on another day, and this time gave them a sports drink slushie to drink and placed ice cold towels on their torsos for 30 minutes beforehand. Not only did the precooling lower their core body temperatures, it also significantly improved their performances. Their heart rates and rates of perceived exertion were lower during the time trial, and they increased their power outputs by 3 percent overall, while improving their total times by 1.3 percent overall.

Try it before your next hot race or ride. Just toss some sports drink in the freezer and dunk a few towels in ice water. You'll not only ride faster but feel better, too.

BREATHE BETTER

The legendary riders in our sport have more than powerful legs. They have tremendous lungs. Take Miguel Indurain, for example. Indurain, who crushed the peloton from 1991 to 1995 for five consecutive Tour de France victories, had an extraordinary lung capacity that allowed him to use 8 liters of oxygen—that's 2 gallons, more than four CamelBak bladders—each minute. That's two liters of pedal-powering oxygen more each minute than his typical competitor, who averages about 6 liters per minute, and twice as much as most of the rest of us.

Obviously, we can increase our oxygen-using capacity simply by training. Hours in the saddle make your heart bigger and stronger, so it can pump more oxygen-rich blood with every beat. Endurance training also creates new capillaries to irrigate working muscles and deliver oxygen where it's needed most. Those adaptations alone can boost the amount of oxygen your body can use by about 10 percent, or another water bottle's worth, each minute you ride.

What many riders don't realize is that while you can't make your lungs larger—that's a fixed factor—you can improve your lung capacity (i.e., maximize what you've got) by training your respiratory strength. To find out just how much, I asked Paul Davenport, PhD, pulmonary researcher and professor at the University of Florida in Gainesville. "You can condition the muscles that support your breathing to make it easier to take deeper breaths and thereby exchange more oxygen in your lungs," he said. In fact, his research found that you can make measurable gains with just a month of consistent training.

In a study of 10 healthy men and women, Davenport found that by blowing into a special "inspiratory muscle trainer" 24 breaths a day, 5 days a week for 4 weeks, the volunteers increased their respiratory muscle strength by 50 percent. That gain probably equals a performance edge of about 2 to 5 percent, said Davenport. "The benefits aren't enormous in the lab. But they're enough to make a difference in a race, where wins happen by seconds."

That said, save your cash and don't bother investing in any of the special lung strengthening devices you see advertised in the backs of magazines. The commercial devices don't match up to what they use in the lab. There are other equally effective ways to strengthen your respiratory muscles, such as the intercostals between your ribs, to promote fuller breathing capability. Here are a few:

BREATHE DEEP . . . THEN DEEPER. World-class triathlete and trainer Eric Harr recommends a breathing exercise that I put to use after breaking some ribs in a bike wreck. (By the way, if you ever find yourself nursing broken ribs, I'd advise you to do the same. Doctors now say it's especially important to maintain respiratory strength during the healing process because you can lose breathing capacity if you baby your ribs with shallow breaths the entire time.)

Breathe in through your nose for 10 seconds, expanding your lungs down and out. When you've fully inhaled, breathe in a little more, then a little more. Challenge yourself to hit maximum lung capacity. Hold that breath for 3 seconds. Exhale slowly out of your mouth to a count of 5 seconds or more. Repeat for 20 breaths.

EXHALE TO EMPTY. You can encourage deeper inhalations by concentrating on full, strong exhalations that fully expel carbon dioxide from your lungs. While riding, try blowing out until you need to inhale. The result will be a fuller, deeper breath.

EXPAND YOUR RIBS. Concentrate on breathing deep into your body, pushing the abdominal part of your lungs down and out. Your abs should expand as much if not more than your chest and you should feel your ribs expand outward.

SWIM LIKE A DOLPHIN. If you're a swimmer, tack on a few "hypoxic" laps to your workout to practice using maximum lung capacity. Take the fullest breath possible, duck underwater, and swim as far as you can without surfacing for air. With practice, you should be able to make it farther and farther across the pool.

PROTECT YOUR AIRBAGS. Lung tissue gets stiffer over the years; with age, you can't inflate as fully and your alveoli pop, giving you less oxygen-exchanging capacity. A little of this, like wrinkles, is inevitable. But much age-related decline is exacerbated by lifestyle factors, says Davenport. "Pollutants like smoke, even from cigars, and air pollution rob our lung capacity more quickly." Protect yourself by avoiding smoke, riding less-trafficked roads, and not riding during high-ozone times such as rush hour on hot summer days.

How do you know if it's all working? Take this test that Harr cooked up to gauge his own breathing improvements.

Start with a 15-minute warmup.

Using a hill that takes about 5 minutes to climb, head up the climb, counting how many breaths (one inhale, one exhale) it takes to reach the top.

Each time you do it, try to do it in fewer breaths.

Harr's personal best is reaching the top in about 25 breaths, or five breaths per minute.

GIVE YOUR MUSCLES A SQUEEZE

Mock the high socks all you want, but compression clothing (socks, shorts, and/or tights), worn both on and off the bike, can help you produce more power. Though studies aimed at finding performance enhancement from wearing compression clothing have yielded mixed results, nearly all the researchers find that the cyclists report feeling fresher and having less muscle soreness when they wear it. Perception, as they say, is reality.

Compression garments apply venous pressure—typically between 10 and 40 millimeters of mercury (mmHg), similar to that applied by an Ace bandage—to encourage blood back to the heart, improve blood oxygen levels, and quicken recovery. Researchers have found that exercisers who wear compression garments during exercise have better muscle oxygenation economy (meaning that their muscles perform ably on less oxygen) and may perform better at threshold exercise levels. Those who wear them after hard efforts have less swelling and muscle damage and improved markers of recovery. Compression also prevents blood from pooling in the lower extremities, which is why so many cyclists wear them when they fly or travel long distances.

Will a pair of compression pants make you bionic? Of course not. But it only makes sense that if you're doing more work with less oxygen and your legs feel fresher and have improved recovery that you're going to be able to train and race faster and harder day after day. I recommend wearing them after hard training days or races, when traveling long distances (especially on a plane), and sleeping in them before a big event (and maybe afterward for quicker recovery). I used to race in my high socks . . . until the International Cycling Union banned them, which could be an indication that compression is a performance enhancer.

RAISE THE BAR

How long can you ride on the drops? If the answer is "only as long as I have to," consider raising your handlebar (a professional bike fit is also a really good idea). Many riders automatically go for the über-pro setup with their handlebars set way below their saddle height. Problem is, they don't actually have the flexibility to reach the drops for any meaningful duration. A higher bar height will open up your torso-to-hip angle, so you have more room to belly breathe and will be less likely to have neck and back pain or saddle discomfort (all of which sap your power). Try positioning your bar evenly at about 1 to 2 inches below the top of the saddle.

TUNE IN

Ever take a silent Spinning class? Nope, I didn't think so. Can you even imagine such a thing? It would be unbearable. I do not advocate riding on the road with music (and I'm not a giant fan of riding on the mountain with it, either, though it's certainly far less risky than being on the road with cars and such). But for training purposes, music can be a powerful performance enhancer. And for the past decade, scientists have been discovering what the iPod army already knew: Music energizes even the most arduous effort. Music and exercise researcher Costas Karageorghis, PhD, of the Brunel University School of Sport and Education in West London explains the power of tunes this way: "Music blocks fatigue and generates feelings of vigor, happiness, and excitement."

Karageorghis and his coworkers found that when men and women listen to music while they work out, they boost their performance (meaning they can go longer and/or faster) by up to 20 percent, which could mean riding 20 miles in the same time it usually takes you to hammer out 17 or 18. When you push the pace and go hard, a little Nine Inch Nails can compel you to pedal harder and faster than you would otherwise as you naturally synchronize your pace to the beat of the music.

Next time you have a hard interval workout on tap, clip on your iPod and hit the trainer (or go to a place you can ride without fear of traffic—and please use one earbud only) and have at it. The music that works best is that which you like best, of course. Researchers have found that commercial dance music tends to provide the optimum 120 to 140 beats per minute for brisk to hard workouts.

SLIP ON THE RIGHT SHADES

Sunglasses to go faster? You bet. There are numerous times I've had to slow down on a ride because I couldn't see well enough to travel comfortably at high speed. Likewise, the right optics can give you the clarity (and confidence) to go really fast.

If you haven't already, pick up a quality pair of cycling-specific shades. Any standard gray- or brown-tint lenses can help reduce visible light and improve vision. But for the best results, pick up a pair with interchangeable lenses. Those multicolored, swappable shades do more than match your jersey and look cool. They offer specialized protection, too. The list below, based on information from sports optometrist Donald Teig, OD, explains how to match the lenses to the conditions.

IF THE AMBIENT LIGHT IS	CHOOSE
Hazy but light (e.g., early morning)	A yellow lens to brighten and clarify
Hazy and overcast	Vermilion (bright red) to brighten vision
Overcast but clear	Clear, antireflective lenses for physical protection
Partly sunny	Light gray lenses for protection without dimming
Very sunny	Dark gray or brown lenses to reduce visible light

Polarized lenses, which are designed to direct scattered light rays into one plane to reduce glare, can help prevent squinting in harsh sunlight, but probably aren't the best choice for cycling. For one, they flatten the terrain, so you can't read contrast, especially in the early morning or evening. You can also miss important road hazards, such as slick oil or water spots, because the lens reduces the glare.

WARM UP ... BUT NOT TOO MUCH

No question: A thorough warmup improves performance. But a recent study comparing a long 50-minute track-racing warmup with an abbreviated 15-minute one found that the longer warmup caused more fatigue and led to less power output than the shortened version. Personally, I found this study a big fat relief. I've long felt that all I needed to be race ready was a quick warmup that hit all the high notes (sent my heart rate up and blew out the pipes, so to speak). More always felt like overkill. But I'd do it anyway, worried I'd somehow fail to perform optimally otherwise.

The science is pretty straightforward. Warming up can help you go faster at the gun by increasing muscle temperature, dilating blood vessels, raising your heart rate, boosting your anaerobic metabolism, and triggering a process called post-activation potentiation (PAP), a biochemical change in your muscle cells that enhances their ability to contract. Problem is, too much warming up can take your muscles from primed to pooped. What to do? I went straight to the source—the study's coauthor Brian R. MacIntosh, PhD, a professor of kinesiology at the University of Calgary.

"The warmup should 'prime the neural circuits,' make the body aware and ready for the task at hand," said MacIntosh. "The goal should be to do a little bit of work at the intensity that you will be using during the competition." How much is enough? Scientists don't yet know, but current thinking is you can keep it brief—try 15 to 20 minutes, including hard surges of 1 to 2 minutes. Your legs should feel open and ready to go (not heavy or tired) when you hit the line.

USE YOUR ANKLES WISELY

Nobody really recommends "ankling" (intentionally flexing and extending the ankle during the pedal stroke) anymore, as it can lead to Achilles tendon problems without producing significantly more power. But, as mentioned in Chapter 1, that doesn't mean you should neglect this essential cycling platform, because strong ankles will help you ride faster. And when your ankles wear out, so do you.

A recent study in the *Journal of Electromyography and Kinesiology* found that when riders fatigue, it's their ankles that give out first, making it nearly impossible to maintain an efficient pedal stroke. The solution: Strengthen your ankles so they provide a rock-steady platform for the long haul. This following technique will get the job done.

Bent-knee heel raise: Stand with your feet parallel and shoulder width apart, knees slightly bent. Raise your heels off the floor as high as you can. Pause, then slowly lower them to the floor. That's one rep; do 3 sets of 15 to 20. As they get easier, try them single-legged.

WEAR SUNSCREEN

This smart skincare advice also can help you keep your speed when the heat is high. The sun saps your energy, especially if it has a chance to cause a sunburn. Sunscreen can help deflect the rays and effectively keeps you cooler, so you have more energy to burn on your bike. Choose a light waterproof and sweatproof spray that provides full coverage and an SPF protection of 15 or higher. I like KINeSYS Sports because it isn't sticky or slippery and allows my skin to breathe.

FAST BODY
Fine-tuning your human frame.

Cyclists spend 20,000 hours on
their bikes and often zero on their
bodies outside of their bikes . . .
That can lead to problems.
—Allison Westfahl, director of personal training
at Flatiron Athletic Club in Boulder, Colorado

Indeed. We're all guilty as charged at some point. We get so focused on riding our bike that we forget about the body that powers that wonderful machine. The result is often subpar performance. Or worse, as in the case of Tom Danielson, who had to pull out of the Tour of California one year because of debilitating back pain from a herniated disc in his L5 region.

When I asked him about it, he described it as a sharp, shooting pain that radiated from his back all the way to behind his knees. "It freaked me out. I felt like I was just shutting down," he said. While the herniation itself could have been a residual injury from a horrific 2007 crash that shattered his shoulder and broke his collarbone, Danielson believes that neglecting his core work as he rehabbed his shoulder opened the door for bigger problems. "I have always done core work in the winter, but with all the physical therapy I was doing to rehab my shoulder, it fell by the wayside," he said. Once he got back on track, the pain subsided and he enjoyed his usual success on the bike. He and Westfahl even wrote a book together about it, aptly titled *Tom Danielson's Core Advantage.*

A strong core is indeed a big advantage, because cycling demands a rock-solid core to provide a platform for pushing into those pedals; strong glutes for holding you steady in the saddle and propelling you down the road; and sheer power for explosive sprints, accelerations, kicking over monster climbs, and launching a well-timed attack. Unfortunately, cycling's tripod position in which the saddle, bar, and pedals support your weight requires core strength but doesn't necessarily develop it. Likewise, pushing pedals may give you bulging quads and diamond-cut calves, but it does little for your glutes, especially your outer glutes, whose job it is to keep you locked down on your saddle.

How's your core strength? Try this little test.

PERFECT PLANK

Prop yourself facedown on the floor with your upper body supported by your forearms, your elbows directly beneath your shoulders. Your torso should be up off the floor so your body is in a straight line, supported by your forearms and toes. Your back should not arch or droop. Hold as long as possible without drooping or arching your back.

How long could you hold it before you started quivering? Fifteen seconds? Thirty? Could you make it 2 minutes? You should be able to hold it at least 60 seconds, but 2 minutes is the gold standard.

Now what about the strength of your stabilizing glute muscles? Try this.

HIP CHECK

In front of a mirror, stand in your bare feet, arms outstretched in front of you, feet about hip width apart. Lift your right foot off the floor in front of the supporting (left) leg. Keeping your body tall, squat down as far as comfortably possible and then return to a standing position. Repeat 3 to 5 times. Switch legs.

Watch your waistband throughout the exercise: It should stay level, not dip to one side or another. Also watch your knees: They should remain aligned, not collapse inward or wobble. Any up-and-down movement of your pelvis or wobbling in your knees indicates weak stabilizing muscles. When you see a rider start to seesaw in the saddle and collapse over the bar, it's a sign that those muscles are flying the white flag. And, for most cyclists, those foundation muscles in the hips and core throw in the towel long before their legs give out.

SNAP TO IT

Cyclists don't just need stability, they need snap—that explosive power that shoots you off the start and helps you bridge gaps, crest climbs, and gun it to the finish. That doesn't mean going to the gym for lots of leg presses. It means training all your big lower body muscles to detonate on demand so you can push a bigger gear faster.

That's why I'm giving you a full chapter on plyometrics—jumping exercises that make your muscles synchronize to exert maximum force faster. The bottom line: If you want to dance on those pedals, you need to perform explosive work off the bike.

How's your lower body power? Get your baseline reading with this long jump test.

Stand with your toes behind a line on the floor, feet somewhere between hip and shoulder width apart. Crouch down and swing your arms backward. Then swing your arms forward and jump forward as far as you can. Land on both feet and mark the spot where your heels hit. (Go ahead and take a couple of practice jumps before giving it your best shot.) You want to hit at least 7 feet 3 inches if you're a man, 5 feet 7 inches if you're a woman. An excellent score would be more than 8 feet for a man or over 6 feet 6 inches for a woman.

The chapters that follow are dedicated to creating a strong, powerful cycling foundation that is ready for anything and resistant to injury. Cycling may be nonimpact, but it's repetitive, which puts stress on your joints, ligaments, muscles, and tendons, and the cartilage that cushions them. One weak link in the chain and you're stalled out. So think of this opening workout plan as making you fit to get fast—really fast. Speaking of fast, I've worked with enough cyclists to know they don't really relish gym time. I don't either. So these workouts cut to the chase. No filler. No fluff. Just the moves you need to feel better on your bike.

Even better: no gym required. That means no excuses for not starting today. Flip the page and let's start at the beginning.

5

Fast Foundation

Strengthen your cycling core for easy speed.

Fast Fact: The average US adult now spends nearly 8 full hours a day—that's 56 hours a week—planted on their seat. The easiest way to increase your speed is to get off your butt and strengthen the powerhouse pelvic muscles of the glutes and hips that you're sitting on.

Two years ago, I started having left knee pain whenever I tried to ride hard, and it would also flare up at random times during the day, such as when I was working the clutch in my car or taking the stairs. I rested, stretched, iced, and popped ibuprofen. Nothing made it go away. Finally I went to see a sports physiatrist, who assured me my knee joint was rock solid and structurally sound. "I think the problem is your glutes," he said as he asked me to lie on my left side with my legs bent and stacked. He put his hands on my outer right leg, midthigh, and told me to push as hard as I could.

"Cake," I thought as I pushed with all my might. "Push!" he barked. "I *am* pushing," I thought, pressing as hard as I could into his hand, but still unable to budge my leg upward against the resistance. "For how strong you are, you should've been able to lift your leg," he said as he finally let go. "Your outer glutes are barely firing. They're so weak, they've probably forgotten how."

Damn. As a writer, I spend a whole lot of time sitting on my strongest muscle. As a cyclist, I was still spending a whole lot of time planted on my engine without doing enough to keep it strong. Now my weakened caboose wasn't just coming along for the ride, it was slowing me down. As I lamented to my go-to sports medicine pro Andy Pruitt, EdD, who works with cyclists of all stripes at the Boulder Center for Sports Medicine in Colorado, he assured me I was far from alone.

"Weak glutes are nearly epidemic, even in cycling circles," he told me. Your glutes provide pelvic stability when you pedal. But cycling uses other muscles more, like those massive quads; so often the glutes just come along for the ride and grow disproportionately weak. When they're weak, you're likely to have more side-to-side motion, especially after a few hours in the saddle. Weak glutes not only make you less solid in the saddle, they also (as yours truly learned the hard way) can contribute to knee pain or injury—a potential nightmare for cyclists, whose knees need to track about 5,400 times each hour. "Many persistent aches and pains in our knees, ankles, feet, and even back begin with weak glutes," said Pruitt.

The good news: Building strong buns as well as a stable core (more on that in a bit) means better stability in the saddle (i.e., no hip rocking) and ultimately a stronger, faster pedal stroke.

THE CYCLIST'S CORE

Here's the deal. By now you've certainly heard about your "core," which depending on who you talk to includes the muscles in your abs, sides, and back. Your abdominals and obliques (the "twisting" muscles at the sides of your trunk) are like a power cord from your arms pulling the bar as you climb and sprint to your legs churning the cranks. They also act as girders that hold your torso stiff, so you have a solid platform to push against and put power into your pedals. When your core fatigues, the force from your pedal stroke sends you bobbing back and forth instead of propelling you forward.

In one study published in the *Journal of Strength and Conditioning Research*, researchers monitored a group of 15 competitive cyclists as they pedaled on a treadmill, holding about 16 mph while the incline increased 1 percent every 3 minutes. A week later, the researchers had the cyclists come back for a retest. Only this time they had them perform a core-muscle-fatiguing workout first. This time when they hopped aboard the treadmill, their pedaling mechanics came undone. Without strong core muscles providing a stable platform, their legs flapped in and out during their pedal stroke. Over time, that kind of sloppy pedaling may not only steal your power but also lead to injury.

So strong abs, back, and obliques are essential for power production. But they aren't the end of the story. The cyclist's core continues down into the glutes and hips. And sitting weakens the entire system. When you sit for extended periods of time, your hip flexors and hamstrings adapt to being balled up by becoming short and tight, while the muscles that support your spine become weak, stretched, and stiff. Unfortunately, the classic cycling position doesn't exactly help matters. Check out your posture sometime while you're tapping away at your computer. Then check your posture while you're spinning down the road. The difference? Some of us may actually be more aero at our desks. Otherwise, not much. And therein lies the problem.

"Cycling puts your legs in a position much like you are at a desk job," says competitive cyclist and chiropractor Ronald DeJong of the

Texas Back Institute. "It also develops your quads while further tightening your hip flexors and hamstrings, which limits your pelvic mobility and can prevent your glutes from firing correctly." This lopsided tug-of-war between the front and back of your body can also lead to tight iliotibial bands and inflammation in your sacro-iliac joints between your hips and the bottom of your back.

Speaking of your back: The classic road cycling position has you bent forward, which stretches out your back muscles (especially if your hips are also tight), while your abdominal muscles hang slack and grow weak. Combine that unsupported, bent-over posture with a pelvis that is pulled forward by tight hamstrings and hip flexors, and you also lose the natural, healthy curvature in your lower back. That not only compromises your pedaling power but also puts you at risk for showstopping back pain because it puts too much pressure on your spine.

Your spine is composed of 24 vertebrae. Between those vertebrae are fluid-filled cushions known as disks. "Imagine your spinal disks as jelly-filled doughnuts," Pruitt told me during our conversation. "When the pressure on them from the top is uniform, the jelly is evenly distributed. When you bend forward, the jelly is pushed back, stressing the skin of that doughnut. If you're sitting all day, that jelly is pressing back there for eight hours. Now toss a leg over a saddle and add another two hours in an even more extreme position, pressing that jelly further and further, until . . . *pop*, out it comes." That's a herniation. In cyclists, it happens most frequently in the lumbar (lower back) region close to the base of the spine, and it can cause a world of pain as that bulging disk presses against the surrounding spinal nerves.

Core work is to your spine what brushing and flossing is to your teeth, said Pruitt, "something you've got to do just to keep what you have." That means strengthening the entire cycling core—abs, obliques, back, hips, and glutes. "Too many cyclists focus on their abs but forget everything else," he said.

THE FLEXIBILITY FACTOR

All the core strength in the world won't improve your pedal stroke unless you have the mobility to go with it. Because pedaling involves a very limited, repetitive range of motion, you never fully contract or extend your legs. Over one season alone that can lead to muscular rigor mortis, especially in your hamstrings, lower back, and glutes, said Pruitt. The result: general aches and pains and genital numbness as your hamstrings yank your pelvis onto the nose of your saddle.

By contrast, improved flexibility lets you save watts wasted to poor on-the-bike position and cycling technique while you gain watts through pure power. "So many cyclists overlook flexibility," said Pruitt. "But flexibility is crucial for proper bike fit. And if you want to be a better time trialist, you'll have much less drag and ride much faster if you're able to bend a couple inches closer to your toes."

When to stretch and how to stretch is nearly as controversial as religion and politics these days. I generally recommend a little traditional 30-second reach-and-hold static stretching in the morning and/or evening, focusing particularly on the quads, glutes, and hamstrings. But I'll be honest, for me personally, stretching often falls by the wayside.

An even better approach that I've found for improving range of motion is to incorporate flexibility moves into your core work, so you strengthen the muscles that are weak and stretch the ones that are tight. I'm a fan of Mark Verstegen's (Core Performance) and Eric Goodman's (Foundation Training) methods. Both have developed exercise systems that create balanced strength and mobility for every sport. Goodman, who has worked with top pro cyclists and has a particular interest in cycling, has seen cyclists improve in just 2 weeks. "By strengthening the posterior chain and improving your range of motion through the hips, you support your spine and allow your glutes to fire more forcefully. When those notoriously tight spots are more supple, you can raise your saddle, sit back, tuck down, and enjoy a more powerful and comfortable ride," says Goodman.

I'm also a fan of regular self-massage to keep your muscles supple and responsive to training in a full, unhindered range of motion. A foam roller (see "Keep on Rolling" on page 70) is a cyclist's best friend between visits to a massage therapist.

THE SPEED PAYOFF

This chapter introduces a cardinal component of getting fast—creating a powerful and stable, yet fluid and mobile, cycling core. The plan is designed to fix imbalances; free your pelvis and spine to fall into a healthy, neutral position; and get your glute muscles firing on all cylinders. The Get Fast! payoff:

➤ *Climb in bigger gears.* Strong core muscles increase your power transfer from your arms to your legs, especially when you're pushing out of the saddle. The stronger you get, the bigger a gear you can push up hills, the faster you can reach the top.

➤ *Sprint like lightning.* Watch the top pro sprinters jackhammering to the finish and you can actually see their core muscles responding to the opposite side pressure as they pedal, sending force back into their legs. A strong cycling core focuses the power of your pedal stroke into a straight line down the road.

➤ *Go the distance.* The stronger your core, the longer you can hammer along without fatigue.

➤ *Conquer 'cross and dirt trails.* Your core stabilizes your bike and body over rough surfaces and helps you pull the front wheel up and over obstacles.

➤ *Stay seated, safely and comfortably.* It's hard to set a PR when your sensitive tissues are going numb and you're standing to stretch every 6 minutes. Ergonomic saddles are one way to lighten the load, but another—and maybe better—way is core strength. "Strong abdominal muscles hold your pelvis back on the saddle where it belongs, keeping weight off those areas," says Pruitt. "When your core muscles are weak or fatigued, your pelvis rocks forward, and that's when you run into trouble with pressure and numbness."

The Get Fast! Cycling Core Plan

The following plan targets cycling core strength and flexibility. One exercise you won't find, though: ab crunches. Cyclists don't need them (nobody does, really). Crunches have you flexing forward over and over again in the same chair- and saddle-centric position. Instead, this plan concentrates on core moves that keep your spine straight while challenging your abs, obliques, back, hips, and glutes.

Perform the routine as a circuit: Do 10 to 15 reps of each exercise, moving immediately from exercise to exercise, without rest. When you're finished, repeat the sequence. Aim to work your core 2 to 3 days a week—even during riding season. Unlike other muscles, your core muscles don't get adequate conditioning from riding alone, so it's important to keep them strong off the bike. Oh, and it's equipment free, so you can do it anywhere, anytime, no excuses. The whole workout will take about 15 minutes.

Good Morning

glutes, hamstrings, and back

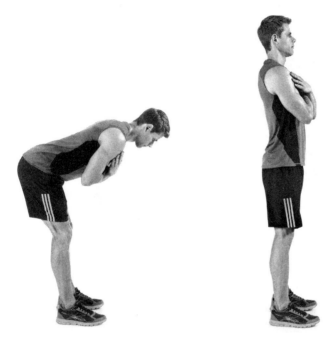

Stand with your legs shoulder width apart, arms across your chest, and press your butt behind you.

Hinge forward at the hips, keeping your chest up and back straight, knees slightly bent, and weight on your heels.

Keeping your spine extended and chest high, pull yourself back up by contracting your glutes and hamstrings. Keep your glute muscles contracted all the way to the top of the movement. Repeat.

Windmill

adductors (inner thighs), back, hamstrings, glutes, and shoulders

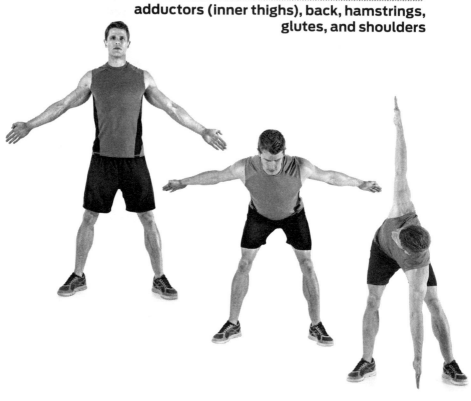

Stand with your legs in a wide straddle stance, knees slightly bent, butt pressed back, chest high, and weight on your heels. Extend your arms in front of you and hold for 15 seconds.

Sweep your arms behind you, palms facing up, squeezing your shoulder blades and contracting your triceps.

Keeping your shoulders back and back flat, hinge forward and reach to the ground with your left hand while reaching to the ceiling with your right, looking up to the right hand. Keep your hips squared; only your torso should twist.

Reverse your twist as you bring your right hand to the floor by your left. Then immediately twist and reach back to the ceiling with your right hand. Repeat for a full set. Then switch sides.

Crank Plank

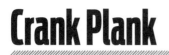

abs, obliques, and shoulders

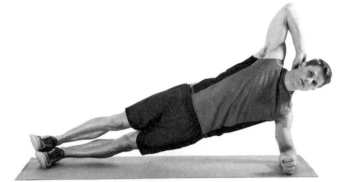

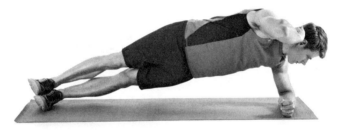

Assume a side plank position, with your left arm extended, elbow on the floor directly beneath your shoulder, feet stacked. Place your right hand behind your head, elbow pointing up.

Keeping your hips stacked, slowly rotate your torso, bringing your right elbow toward your left arm.

Rotate to the starting position. Repeat for a full set. Then switch sides.

Single-Leg Bridge

hamstrings, glutes, and hip flexors

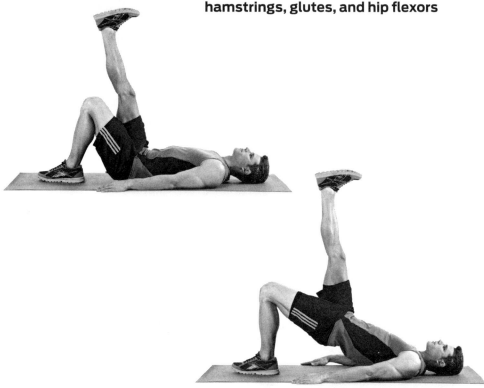

Lie back on the floor with your knees bent 90 degrees and feet flat. Extend your right leg, keeping your knees in line.

Push into your left foot and press your hips into the air so your body forms a straight line from your shoulders to your bent knee.

Return to the starting position. Repeat for a full set. Then switch sides.

Spider-Man Pushup

abs, obliques, shoulders, chest, and arms

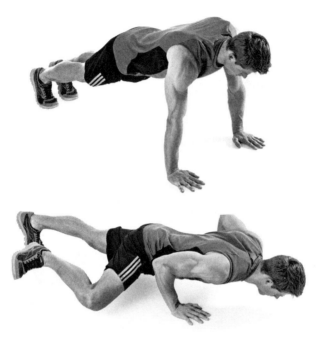

Assume a plank position, with your arms extended, palms flat beneath shoulders, and legs extended, feet flexed. Keep your abs tight.

Bend your arms, lowering your chest toward the floor. At the same time, bend your right leg out to the side, bringing your right knee toward your right elbow.

Pause, then return to the starting position. Switch sides. Repeat for a full set, alternating sides throughout.

Scorpion

**back and glutes;
also stretches chest, hips,
shoulders, and back**

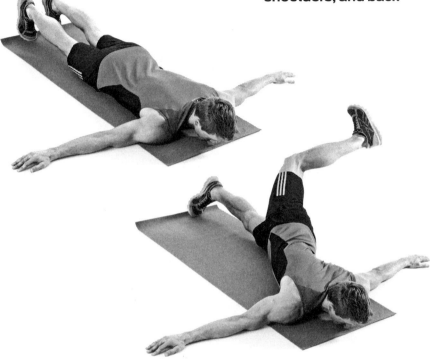

Lie facedown with your arms out to the sides, shoulders flat on the floor.

Lift your right leg off the floor and, twisting your torso, reach it across the back of your body as far as possible toward your left hand.

Return to the starting position. Repeat to the other side. Repeat for a full set to each side, alternating sides throughout.

Single-Leg Stepdown

glutes, quads, and hamstrings

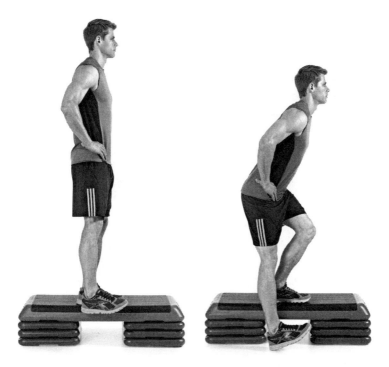

Place your hands on your hips and stand on a 12- to 18-inch step with only your left foot on top of the step, allowing the other leg to hang in the air.

Pull your navel toward your spine and, keeping your chest lifted, slowly step down with your right foot and gently tap your right heel on the floor.

Keeping your left heel firmly planted on the step, return to the starting position. Repeat for a full set. Then switch sides.

Tipping Bird

hamstrings, hips, and glutes

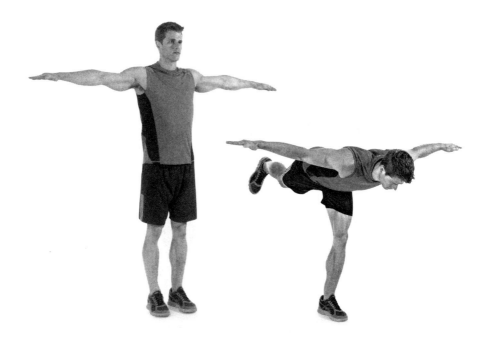

Stand tall with your arms out to the side at shoulder height.

Keeping your right leg extended, lift your right foot behind you and balance on your left leg.

Slowly hinge forward from the hips, tipping your torso forward toward the ground while extending your right leg straight behind you, foot flexed, until your body forms a straight line from your head to your heel. Stop when you're parallel to the floor.

Return to the starting position. Switch sides. Alternate for a set of 10 on each side.

Ball Mountain Climber

TARGETS:

abs, back, obliques, and hips

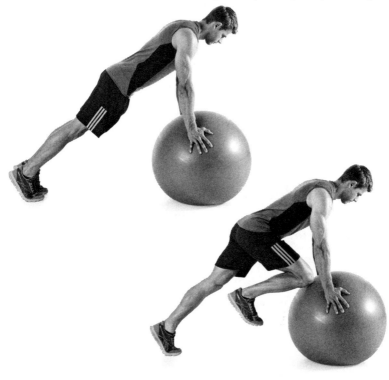

Assume the pushup position with your hands on the sides of an exercise ball. Contract abs for support.

Lift one foot off the floor and pull that knee toward your chest.

Return to the starting position and repeat with the other leg. That's one rep. Continue alternating sides for 10 to 12 on each side.

Keep on Rolling

Like a cable that's been crimped one too many times, our hardworking muscles eventually develop kinks—small adhesions or knots that make you stiff and sore, preventing you from pedaling with full, unhindered mobility and power. A massage therapist can rub them out. But most of us don't have the luxury of a massage every day or even every week. You do if you have a foam roller.

These pressed cylinders allow you to keep your muscles healthy and supple yourself, says Scott Levin, MD, sports medicine specialist at Somers Orthopaedic Surgery and Sports Medicine Group in Carmel, New York. "Rolling along these rollers provides myofascial release [breaks adhesions and scar tissue within the muscle and fascia that covers the muscle], warms and stretches the muscles, and increases circulation," says Levin. "It's convenient and very effective because it allows you to home in on your problem spots and work them to your comfort level. Done after a hard workout or ride, rolling also can prevent delayed onset muscle soreness." I agree. I think it's the perfect finish to a hard plyo session. I also find it's a perfect start and finish to a day planted on your posterior.

The best part about foam roller work is that it releases areas you might not have even known were bound. Last year, during a continuing education session in New York, I noticed as I sat there for a few hours in the hard chairs that my hips were feeling achy. I fidgeted and shifted my weight and stretched a bit in my seat. Then, thankfully, the presenter invited us all to grab a foam roller from the corner of the room and find a spot on the floor. The first move he had us do was an adductor massage, where we positioned ourselves face-down with our adductor draped over the roller and massaged upward toward the groin muscle, settling our weight into the roller.

I thought I was going to hit the ceiling. Turns out my violin-string tight adductors and groin muscles were pulling on the abductors and outer glutes, causing a world of discomfort. I rolled out the kinks and spent the rest of the day ache and pain free. As a cyclist, you'll find tight, knotted spots throughout your lower body, but especially through your iliotibial (IT) bands. Follow these directions, slowly rolling back and forth over the targeted muscle group about 10 to 12 times.

If a spot feels tender, hold the roller there and press your weight into it, then roll through it until it feels better. You can roll daily or even several times daily, but aim for at least two or three times a week to keep your muscles supple.

Calves

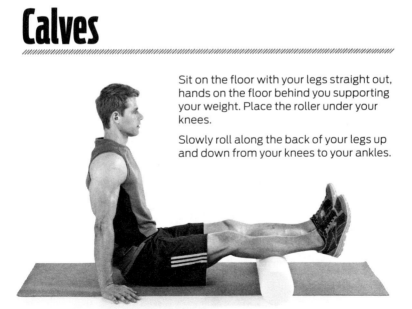

Sit on the floor with your legs straight out, hands on the floor behind you supporting your weight. Place the roller under your knees.

Slowly roll along the back of your legs up and down from your knees to your ankles.

Hamstrings

Sit with your right leg on the roller; bend your left knee and put your hands on the floor behind you.

Roll up and down from your knee to just under your right butt cheek.

Switch legs.

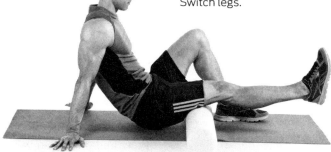

Quads

Lie facedown on the floor and place the roller under your hips.

Lean on your right leg.

Roll up and down from your hip to your knee.

Switch legs.

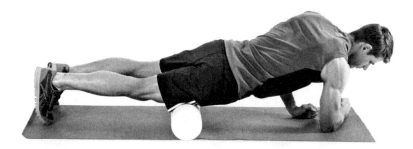

IT Band

Lie on your side with the roller placed just below the hip. Bend your top leg and place that foot in front of your body for balance and to control the pressure on the roller.

Roll down along the outside of the leg from the hip to the knee and back again.

Switch legs.

Butt

Sitting on the foam roller, cross your right leg over your left knee and lean toward your right hip, putting your weight on your hands for support.

Slowly roll one butt cheek over the roller.

Switch sides.

Back

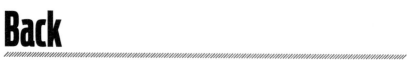

Sit on the floor with the foam roller behind you. Lace your fingers behind your head and lean your upper back onto the roller.

Tighten your abs and glutes and slowly move up and down the roller.

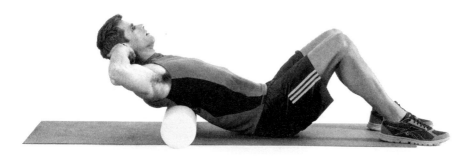

Adductor

Assume a plank position on the floor, supporting yourself on your elbows and forearms. Bend your right leg and drape your leg over the roller so it is parallel to your body with the roller resting against your groin muscles.

Sink your weight into the roller and roll along the length of your adductor to your bent knee and back again.

Switch sides.

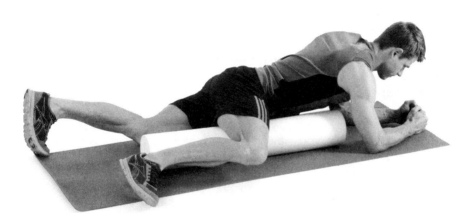

Stand Up

A survey of more than 6,300 men and women in the United States reported that we now spend nearly 8 eight hours a day—that's 56 hours a week—planted on our behinds. Before you dismiss that statistic as something that only applies to all those sedentary folks out there, take a little mental poll.

How long do you spend behind a desk all day? And behind the steering wheel of a car? And on the sofa? Even if you manage to ride 150 miles a week, unless you have a job that keeps you moving, I'm going to venture that most of your nonriding time is chair time. I know it is for me (a writer by trade) and for many of the cyclists I work with.

Blame that computer you're tapping away on. Electronic living has all but sapped every flicker of activity from our daily lives. You can shop, pay bills, make a living, and, thanks to social media, even catch up with friends without ever so much as standing up.

But you ride, right? So you're not sedentary. Don't bet on it, says Genevieve Healy, PhD, of the University of Queensland in Australia, who has coined the term *active couch potato* to describe regular exercisers who sit too much (including, she admits, herself). Many of us are so sedentary during the day that the hour we spend on our bikes is not enough to counteract the harmful effects of 8, 9, maybe 10 hours of sitting. If you can't lose your gut, lower your cholesterol, or get your blood sugar under control despite your regular rides, chair time may be to blame.

In a recent study of 168 volunteer men and women, Healy and her coworkers reported that regardless of how much (or how little) moderate to vigorous exercise the volunteers did, those who took more breaks from sitting had slimmer waists, lower body mass indexes, and healthier body fat and blood sugar levels than those who sat the most.

In a recent lifestyle study of 17,000 men and women, Canadian researchers cut right to the chase: The longer you spend sitting, the more likely you are to die an early death no matter how fit you are.

"Sitting for an extended period of time causes your body to shut down at the metabolic level," explains Marc T. Hamilton, PhD, professor at the Pennington Biomedical Research Center in Baton Rouge, Lousiana. When your muscles, especially the large ones in your legs, are immobile, your circulation slows dramatically. So you use less of your blood sugar and you burn far less fat. Hamilton's research shows that key fat-burning enzymes—such as lipoprotein lipase (LPL)—that are responsible for breaking down triglycerides in your bloodstream simply start switching off when you sit too long. Sit for a full day and you can expect LPL activity to plummet by 50 percent.

As if all that isn't bad enough, circulation in your legs is reduced by two-thirds while you sit, causing blood to pool in your calves, which slows your recovery from hard workouts and leaves you feeling sluggish when it's finally time to ride. Improve your health and your cycling performance by standing up as often as possible on the job. A few tips:

Take the long way. You have to get up sometime to grab some water or use the restroom. Take the long way around the building, use the stairs, stretch your legs, and so forth for 5 minutes before returning to your desk. Repeat five times a day.

Request a convertible desk. A few of my editors at *Bicycling* and *Men's Health* magazines swear by these, and I've seen them popping up as options at other companies. Ask your human resources department if they offer stand-up workstations (especially if you have a history |of back pain). These convertible desks allow you to raise your work surface to standing height. Those I know who try them leave them up all day.

Walk and talk. Rather than meeting a colleague to brainstorm around a table in a stuffy conference room, grab a pen and pad and walk and talk.

Take a stand. Take and return all your phone calls on your feet. If space permits, pace a little while you converse.

6

Fast-Firing Muscles

Put explosive power in your legs.

Fast Fact: Between ages 50 and 80, we can lose about half (yes, half!) of the muscle fibers in our thighs unless we do something to stop the slide. Sadly, the first to go are the snappy, fast-twitch type II variety that we need for speed, but that go largely untouched on long, slow rides.

I've had an on-and-off love affair with the weight room. About 15 years ago, I pushed iron faithfully, following a periodic schedule that included heavy doses of leg presses, squats, hamstring curls . . . the works. I got stronger, yes. But—and I know I'll take heat for saying this—I also got bulkier, to the point where an old roadie, coach, and friend of mine called me a "little gorilla on the bike." Nice.

I wouldn't have minded the hypertrophy if it weren't for the heaviness. I had more strength, but I also had more weight. They weren't really making magic together on the bike (especially on climbs or during sudden accelerations) the way I'd hoped. So I stopped lifting and rode more instead. That worked for a stretch. After a full season, however, I ended up feeling weaker—both on and off my wheels. Determined that there must be a happy medium, I went in search of a sweet spot: a way to get more power into my pedals without unwanted weight. I found it in explosive power training such as plyometrics.

Latin for "measurable increases," plyometrics delivers just that to your muscles. Based on jumping, leaping, and other explosive moves, plyometrics condition your muscles to detonate on demand so you have the split-second force you need to crank up steep inclines, power through rolling terrain, and sprint to the finish line. And they work fast, too. Research shows that a twice-weekly plyometric routine can boost your power endurance (your muscles' ability to contract at near-max force) by 17 percent and increase your lactate threshold cycling power (the max power you can sustain for about an hour) by 3.5 percent in just 4 weeks.

This makes good sense for cyclists for whom power is more important than sheer brute strength. Stuart Phillips, PhD, professor of kinesiology at McMaster University in Hamilton, Ontario, explains it well. "When cyclists push on the pedals, the force they exert is generally a very small percentage of their maximal strength. Riding flat terrain at one hundred rpm is likely one to three percent of maximal force. That's why you can cycle for four to five hours!" says Phillips. Though climbing takes a higher percentage, it's still fairly small. So yes, you need strength to push those gears. But more important for going fast is power—how quickly you can spin those gears and keep them spinning. That's where plyometrics comes in.

MORE POWER TO YOU

To fully appreciate the power of plyometrics, you need to take a brain's-eye view of your muscles. Every muscle in your body consists of fibers that are bundled together in motor units activated by your brain. Large muscles like your thighs have thousands of fibers per unit. Being naturally conservative, your brain will use only the number of motor units it needs for any given job. Moderate efforts in the weight room or on the bike activate some of those motor units, but many, especially those that serve your fast-twitch type II (speed and power) fibers go untouched. Left unused, many of the neurons that once served fast-twitch muscles get rewired to serve their slower counterparts. Others simply die off. That's bad. Especially if you're a master cyclist. Because unless you do something to stop the decline, those neurons start disappearing at a precipitous rate in later adulthood.

That's something Phillips says happens far too often, even among people who exercise. "Someone doing traditional dumbbell squats with ten-pound dumbbells is probably activating zero type II muscle fibers," he explains. The only way to preserve them is by activating them with intensity. Plyometrics jolts them back into action, training your body to recruit maximum motor units with every explosive move. It also works fast. "Our research shows that your muscles respond to a challenge like explosive exercise after just one bout," says Phillips.

Explosive training also makes your muscles faster by training them to use every ounce of potential energy you create when you load them up during the eccentric part of a contraction. Think of your legs as a pair of springs. When you bend into a deep squat, you are stretching out those springs and loading them for action. When you explode up into a jump (as you do in a plyometric jump squat), you are tapping into that potential energy. Plyometric moves are done quickly and explosively over and over, which trains your muscles to stretch and shorten over and over at high speed. So you're increasing not only the number of motor units you're using but also the speed at which you can recruit them, without wasting a drop of energy. This transformation is also quick. Research shows you can increase your fast-twitch firing rates after just one week of training.

Now consider that power is defined as the amount of work done with respect to time. When your muscles are trained to use more fibers and contract at a rapid-fire pace, you can push a bigger gear, turn the cranks more quickly, and go farther down the road in less time. Traditional strength training doesn't necessarily make you faster. Plyometrics does. And you know what else? You don't just gain speed, you also gain endurance. The more motor units you can trigger, the more your brain has at its disposal during hard efforts, and the longer you can go before you fatigue.

More power isn't the only way plyos help you go fast. They also may help you lose unwanted weight (or at least keep you from gaining it) by burning more calories than traditional training. When researchers at Ball State University in Muncie, Indiana, pitted traditional slow reps against high-speed explosive reps during squat exercises, they found that subjects who performed springy, split-second reps burned 11 percent more calories than those doing the same move more slowly. That adds up to 10 to 15 calories, which may not sound like much, but remember that's just for one exercise. Multiply that over a full body workout and you could burn an extra 100+ calories—what you'd burn by running a mile—*and* finish up faster to boot. That doesn't even include the bonus afterburn, the calories you burn when you're done, which the researchers found was boosted by an additional 5 percent with high-speed strength training. Since lean muscle tissue stokes your resting metabolism, all this fast-twitch preservation will also help keep pounds away, especially at midlife, when muscle loss and metabolism meltdown leads to weight gain.

Given all the speed, weight, and power rewards, it's no surprise that Lance Armstrong was spied doing plyometrics along his comeback trail in 2009 (likely under the guidance of his power coach

Peter Park, though other cycling coaches such as Chris Carmichael recommend them as well).

READY, SET, GO!

The following routine contains plyometric moves to power up your hips, glutes, and legs, as well as fire up your core and the support muscles in your torso (especially important for 'cross and off-road riders).

Proper form and technique is essential. Warm up thoroughly for at least 10 minutes. *Always* land softly by recoiling your joints like a spring immediately as you hit the ground. If fatigue is making your form sloppy, stop. Plyometrics work best when you practice quality, not quantity. This workout also assumes you have a foundation of strength. If you've been doing zero strength work, first prep your muscles and strengthen your connective tissues with 4 to 6 weeks of traditional squats, lunges, stepups, and pushups before you begin.

Finally, for the best results, combine this plyo routine with high-intensity sprint work on the bike (the trainer obviously works best here). Put the finishing touches on this workout with 1 to 3 sets of 5 30-second sprints. Warm up your legs with some Spinning. Then throw it in a bigger gear, jump out of the saddle to get the sprint going, and sit and crank for 30 seconds. Recover in an easy gear for 30 seconds and repeat. Take about 5 minutes to recover between sets. End each workout with a very light, high-cadence cooldown.

The Get Fast! Plyo Workout

Do 1 to 2 sets of the prescribed reps, resting 1 minute between sets. Do the routine twice a week, allowing at least a day off between workouts. Plyometrics are best done to rebuild in the off-season. Wrap them up by the end of March, or whenever you start doing more on-the-bike intensity and racing.

Warmup Swings

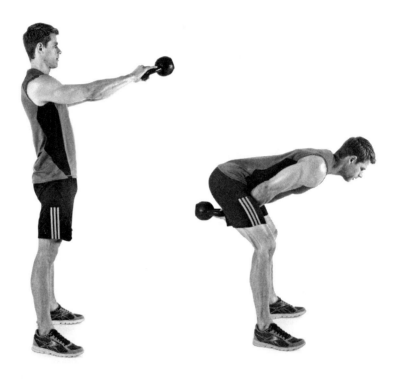

Stand with your feet wide apart, holding a relatively light kettlebell with both hands, arms hanging down in front of you. (You can also use a medicine ball.)

Keeping your back straight, squat back, pressing your hips way back and swinging the kettlebell between your legs and behind your hips.

Stand up, pressing your hips forward and swinging the weight up just past chest level.

Do 10 to 15 reps.

Jump Squat

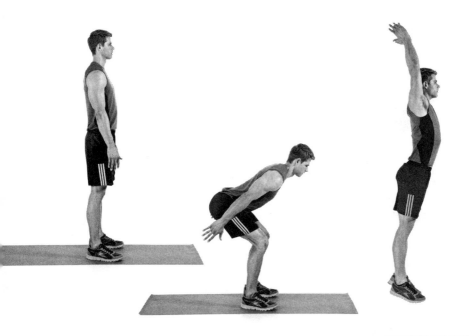

Stand with your feet shoulder-width apart, arms at your sides.

Sit back into a squat, lowering your hips until your thighs are parallel to the floor.

Jump up as explosively as you can while reaching for the ceiling.

Land gently, and immediately lower into another squat. Start with 10 jumps. Work up to 20.

Side Hops

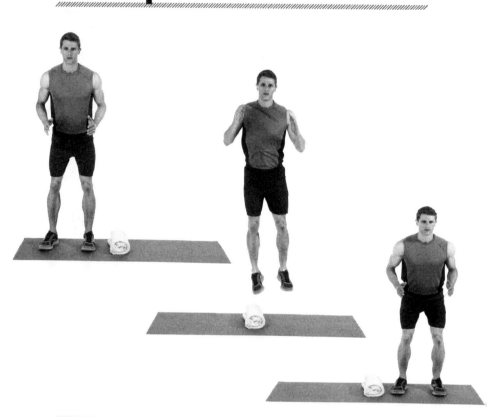

Place a rolled-up towel on the floor and stand next to it.

Bend your knees and jump up and sideways over it.

As you land, immediately bend at the knees again and jump right back to the starting position.

Start with 10 jumps. Work up to 20.

Pedaling Split Jump

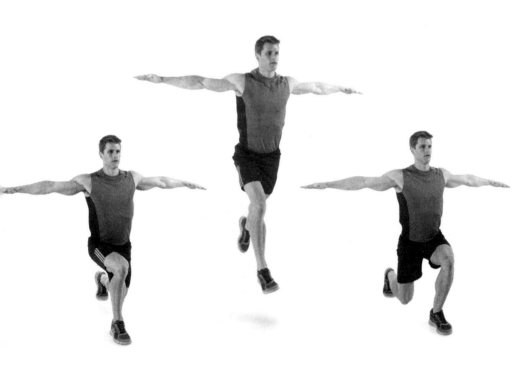

Stand with your right leg forward and your left leg back behind you. Bend your right knee and dip your left knee toward the floor, so you're in a lunge position. Place your arms out to the sides.

Swiftly jump up and switch legs, driving the back knee up (like the upward pedal stroke) as you bring it forward.

Softly land in a lunge position and immediately jump again.

Start with 10 jumps. Work up to 20.

Ovation Pushup

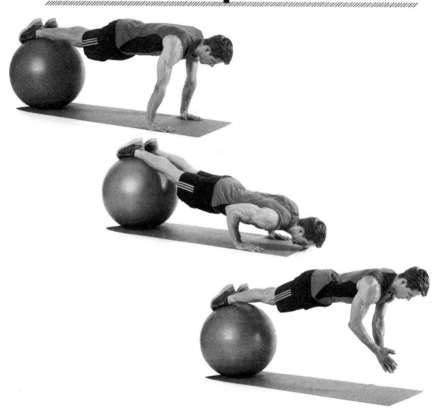

Lie facedown on an inflated exercise ball with both hands on an exercise mat or cushioned surface. Walk hands out until the ball is under your thighs or shins. Position your hands directly below your shoulders.

Keeping your torso straight, bend your elbows and lower your chest toward the floor until your arms are bent 90 degrees.

Push up as hard as you can, clap your hands once, and return to the starting position, before immediately dropping into another repetition.

Start with 6 to 8 reps. Work up to 10 to 12.

No ball? You can do this on the floor, but it's much harder.

Blastoff

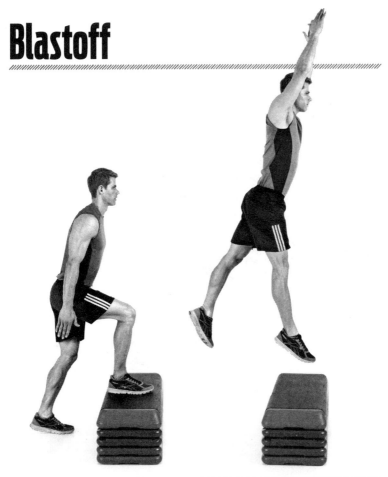

Stand facing a step about 12 to 18 inches high. Plant your right foot on the step.

Forcefully push off your right foot and jump straight up, swinging your arms forward and up for added momentum.

Land with your right foot on the step and immediately push off for the next rep.

Complete a set, and then switch legs. Start with 6 to 8 jumps per leg. Work up to 10 to 12.

7

Fast Frame (Yours!)

Power-to-weight ratio is a two-sided equation. Here's how to find and maximize yours.

Somewhere along the line, cyclists began developing a "you can never be too skinny" mentality. I know some already gaunt and hollowed-out Cat 2s who would cut off their earlobes if it were socially acceptable just to shave off another couple grams. To them I present my teammate Jesse Kelly.

Jesse is a 40-something competitive cyclist who races mountain bikes and tackles long road sportives—such as the Exmoor Beast

Cycle Challenge in England—that take him over 10,000 feet in 100 miles. He's about 5 feet 10 inches tall, 194 pounds, and rides an ancient Bianchi Volpe cyclocross bike he found on Craigslist (complete with a dropper seatpost). The bike squeaks and pings like a mouse caught in a tin can. And this guy is the bane of our annual Team CF (Cystic Fybrosis) charity ride—Cycle for Life. Why? Because when the road tilts skyward 8 to 10 percent and the pack starts sliding backward, Jesse defies all reason and powers his way to the top—while skinny guys in full team kits shake their heads and swear, unable to keep up.

Cycling is a power-to-weight sport, meaning simply that the fastest guys can produce the most power per pound. The problem is that too many riders become absolutely fixated on tinkering with the backside of that equation, while giving little more than a passing nod to developing—really developing—the first half. As mentioned in the previous chapter, power is simply distance traveled over time—getting from point A to point B more quickly. Take a look at any given group of accomplished cyclists, from sprinters to climbers to crit specialists, and you'll quickly see that although dropping extra baggage will help speed you up, you don't have to get skinny to get fast.

That's right, you don't have to be stick-figure thin to be a great rider. "Cyclists need to remember that even pro riders don't maintain those ridiculously lean profiles for more than two or three weeks at a time," says Hunter Allen, power training expert and coauthor of *Cutting-Edge Cycling.* "You really can be too skinny. Especially for everyday riders, there's a point in the power-to-weight equation where you start going in the opposite direction. Riders start getting sick because their immunity is so compromised, and if you lose muscle, your power-to-weight ratio will go down." The goal is finding the sweet spot where you can ride strong and fast, yet be healthy and happy, too.

Your personal sweet spot depends on myriad factors including your height, frame size (yours, not your bike's), body type, and the type of riding you do. With the help of Allen, master coach Joe Friel, and the crack squad at *Bicycling* magazine, we developed this four-step Ideal Cycling Weight Decoder to help you determine a perfect weight you can live, ride, and even race with for life.

Important note: Not every cyclist will need to perform each step. If you ride primarily for recreation and just have a few pounds to lose, the first two or three steps are all you need. If you're already a competitive racer who trains hard and aspires to achieve an optimal racing weight, the entire process will give you that number. Just note that, as Allen mentions above, racing weight is not necessarily a healthy weight to maintain year-round.

STEP 1: CALCULATE YOUR BASELINE WEIGHT

The first step is determining your base weight. Here's how:

To determine your healthy base body weight, use the following formula (and note that this number will need to be adjusted based on your frame size in Step 2).

WOMEN*		MEN	
100 pounds for the first 5 feet of height	➕ 5 pounds for each additional inch	106 pounds of body weight for the first 5 feet of height	➕ 6 pounds for each additional inch
For example, if you're 5 feet 6 inches, your ideal weight is 130 lbs. (100 + 30)		For example, if you're 5 feet 10 inches, your ideal weight is 166 lbs. (106 + 60)	
		Baseline weight	

*Women vary more by height and frame size than men do and therefore have more variation in this ratio.

STEP 2: FACTOR IN YOUR FRAME SIZE

Big boned has become somewhat of a snarky phrase meaning "fat." But it's legit. Just as mountain bike frames come in small, medium, and large, so do our skeletal frames. That's why there's a large range of medically recommended weights for any given height. The best measurement of frame size is your wrist circumference in relation to your height. Measure your wrist with a tape measure and use the following chart to determine whether you are small, medium, or large boned.

	WOMEN*		MEN	
Height under 5'2"	Small = wrist size less than 5.5"		**Height over 5'5"**	Small = wrist size 5.5" to 6.5"
	Medium = wrist size 5.5" to 5.75"			Medium = wrist size 6.5" to 7.5"
	Large = wrist size over 5.75"			Large = wrist size over 7.5"
Height 5'2" to 5'5"	Small = wrist size less than 6"		Adjust your baseline: The baseline weight in the first step is based on a medium frame. For a small body frame, subtract 10%. For a large frame, add 10%.	
	Medium = wrist size 6" to 6.25"			
	Large = wrist size over 6.25"			
Height over 5'5"	Small = wrist size less than 6.25"			
	Medium = wrist size 6.25" to 6.5"			
	Large = wrist size over 6.5"		**Your frame adjusted number***	

*Women vary more by height and frame size than men do and therefore have more variation in this ratio.

Note: Standard body weight formulas are based on averages, which means that results for some people may be slightly skewed. If the number you calculate feels off, either too high or too low, be sure to move on to the next step, which factors in body composition.

STEP 3: FIGURE IN YOUR BODY COMPOSITION

The numbers on the scale don't paint the complete picture of your fitness without more context. You may be at the high end of your weight range but be able to see every sinew of your dense muscular pistons. Likewise, the scale may say 150, but you have the muscle tone of . . . well maybe not so much muscle tone. That's why it helps to know your body composition—a set of percentages that breaks down your weight into percent fat and lean pedal-pushing muscle.

Body fat ranges for optimal health are 18 to 30 percent for women (who naturally have more fat) and 10 to 25 percent for men. Athletes tend to have lower fat percentages, with women coming in around 12 to 22 percent and men carrying anywhere from 5 to 13 percent. Don't get too hung up on trimming every little ounce. If you're at the lower end of the spectrum for general fitness, upper end for athletes, you're not going to gain speed by focusing on fat loss. And you might just make yourself sick, says Allen.

"Having a bit more body fat is better for your immune system and consistency on the bike. Once you start pushing too far into the lower ranges, the immune system compromises are great," says Allen. "For men, if you can get down around ten percent, you're in good shape. For women, a good benchmark is eighteen percent."

You can measure your body fat with a special body composition scale (Tanita is a popular brand), available at most box stores. Follow the directions carefully. The reading is sensitive to hydration levels as well as menstruation for women. Like weight, the number will fluctuate, so focus on your average.

Ideal Weight Based on Body Composition

Follow these steps to determine your ideal weight based on body composition.

STEP 1: FIGURE OUT HOW MANY POUNDS OF BODY FAT YOU HAVE

[ ] + [ ] = [ ] lb.

Your current weight · Your body fat percentage · *(i.e, 200 lb. x 0.28 = 56 lb.)*

STEP 2: NEXT, FIGURE OUT YOUR LEAN BODY MASS

[ ] X [ ] = [ ] lb.

Your current weight · Pounds of body fat · *(i.e., 200 lb. - 56 lb. = 144 lb.)*

STEP 3: SUBTRACT YOUR GOAL BODY-FAT PERCENTAGE FROM 1.00

1.00 − [ ] = [ ]

Your goal body fat percentage · *(i.e., 1.00 - 0.20 = 0.80)*

STEP 4: DIVIDE YOUR LEAN BODY MASS BY YOUR ANSWER TO STEP 3

[ ] + [ ] = [ ] lb.

Lean body mass · Answer to Step 3 · *(i.e., 144 lb./0.80 = 180 lb.)*

Your target ideal weight based on body composition [ ] lb.

STEP 5: CALCULATE YOUR TOP COMPETITIVE WEIGHT.

Time to circle around to include that most essential part of this whole equation: power. The single best measure of your cycling performance is your power-to-weight ratio. This figure refers to the maximum power output—measured in watts—that you can sustain for an extended period of time, generally 30 minutes or more.

Joe Friel, who created the Training Bible series, has calculated that top male riders generally carry in the range of 2.1 to 2.4 pounds per inch; top women carry 1.9 to 2.2 pounds per inch. (This ratio isn't the same as your power-to-weight ratio—see "Power Numbers" on page 98—which is considered the gold standard for determining your most competitive cycling weight. But it's close, and it doesn't require an expensive power meter to figure out.)

For elite climbing specialists, those numbers drop, as weight becomes more of a consideration as the pull of gravity increases up those 10 percent grades. Top elite male climbers (we're talking Tour pros here) generally have less than 2 pounds of body weight per inch of height, and elite women have about 1.8 or less pounds per inch. That means a 5 foot 10 inch man would need to weigh in at 140 pounds, and a 5 foot 5 inch woman would need to tip the scales at 117.

There are exceptions, says Friel. Most famously Lance Armstrong, who came in at about 2.1 pounds per inch, but also produced more power. You'll also note that some riders, such as Tour winner Cadel Evans, are just built bigger than Andy or Frank Schleck (see "Body Build" on page 97), but it doesn't make them slower. If you tend toward the muscular side, it can be unrealistic (if not downright counterproductive) to try to drop down to an unnaturally light weight.

Use the ranges above to see how close your goal or current weight is to a weight that would maximize your ability to compete (assuming you have the corresponding fitness). If your goal or current

Body Build

Similar to frame size, most of us can slot our overall build into one of three general categories (recognizing that there are a wide variety of shapes and sizes even within these categories).

Type 1—ectomorph: You tend to be long limbed and not particularly muscular.

Type 2—mesomorph: You are muscular and tend to be proportionally built.

Type 3—endomorph: You are generally more heavyset.

Muscle tissue is dense, so someone who is muscular is always going to be heavier than someone who is less so. But, as you might have guessed, they may also have more horsepower, says James Herrera of Performance Driven Coaching in Colorado Springs, Colorado. "Performance on the bike isn't all about a number on a scale. You've got to have strength to push the gear, leg speed to turn it over, aerobic development to sustain your pace, and optimal body weight so power-to-weight ratio is optimized," he says.

What does that mean in terms of your body type? If you're an ectomorph, you might have a low scale number, but still not maximum strength. Getting in the gym for some squats and leg presses could develop that strength and inch the scale a bit higher, but with positive, not negative, results. Endomorphs need to keep body mass in check. Your muscle is your engine, but you don't need chest and arm muscles like a linebacker to turn cranks. Too much muscle literally weighs you down. While you shouldn't seek to deliberately lose muscle, you may want to avoid gaining it where you don't need it, as in your upper body.

Your type:_____

weight is less than your competitive weight, go back to Step 3 to make sure your body fat is within a healthy range. If it's not, hit the gym to put on lean muscle tissue, and be sure you're properly fueling during and especially after your rides so you don't go into a catabolic state and eat into your precious muscle stores. Be especially sure to

Power Numbers

If you own a power meter (or you plan to make the investment soon), you can get an excellent portrait of your power. Of course, everyone who tries a power meter wants to know the same thing: How many watts can I crank out? But that's not always indicative of your cycling ability. A BMX racer can send the meter soaring upward of 1,500 watts for 5 to 10 seconds. But can he hang for 100-K and do it at the end of a race? Maybe. Maybe not. Here are tests to give you a portrait of your power. Remember to always warm up for 20 minutes first.

Max power: Okay, get it out of your system. Warm up 15 to 20 minutes. Then ride all out for 5 minutes. Recover fully. Repeat 2 to 3 times. Take your best max power.

Your number: _____

Power-to-weight ratio (i.e., holy grail): Find a long hill and perform a 20-minute ascending time trial(TT). If you don't have a hill at your disposal, you can do a 20-minute TT on a flat road or even on the trainer, but try to avoid rolling roads as they will lower your overall power average. Record the average wattage you produced. Then take your morning body weight (calculate it in kilograms by dividing your weight in pounds by 2.2) and divide it into the average watts you produced. So if you weigh 180 pounds (82 kg) and you averaged 270 watts, your power-to-weight ratio is 3.3 watts per kg.

To score a top spot a professional racing team, that number would need to be 6 to 7 watts per kg. Beginner cyclists usually pull in the range of 2.5 to 3.2 for men and 2.1 to 2.8 for women. Fast recreational riders crank out wattages in the range of 3.7 to 4.4 for men and 3.2 to 3.8 for women. To be competitive in 30- to 60-minute time trials, men need to push it above the 4.5 range, and women should come in closer to 4.

Your number: _____

Lactate threshold power (LTP): Here's your breaking point. Above this wattage, your body produces lactic acid faster than you can clear it and you pop. This number is about 40 watts below max—where you can do a 40-K TT. There are various ways to test LTP. Pros determine it in the lab with blood lactate testing. You can do a "poor man's" LTP test with this drill that was popularized by Carmichael Training Systems. Warm up and then ride 8 minutes at the highest power you can maintain. Rest 10 minutes. Repeat. The highest average power of the two tests is your LTP.

Another similar test that is popular now (thanks to power training coach Hunter Allen) is functional threshold power (FTP). Similar to LTP, this is the wattage that you can produce for 1 hour without fatiguing. Coaches like FTP because it's relevant to nearly all cyclists, regardless of the type of riding or racing they do. You can attain that number by performing a 60-minute TT, of course. But that's not really practical for a lot of riders (stop signs, etc., get in the way). An easier method that Allen recommends is performing a 20-minute TT

and multiplying that average wattage by 0.95, since your hour-long wattage would be about 5 percent lower.

Your number: _____

Total picture: Power training gurus such as Andrew Coggan, PhD, coauthor of *Training and Racing with a Power Meter,* like to get a complete picture by indexing efforts at intervals of 5 seconds, 1 minute, 5 minutes, and 20 minutes. "These intervals best reflect neuromuscular power [determined by muscle size and speed and nervous system responsiveness], anaerobic capacity, VO_2 max, and lactate threshold, respectively," he says. Power output over these target durations correlates well with more direct measurements of these different physiological abilities, he says. So it's another way of tracking your strengths and weaknesses as your training progresses.

To see how you're progressing, repeat these tests again after 8 to 12 weeks of training.

meet your daily protein requirements by including protein in every meal and snack.

WORK ONE SIDE AT A TIME

Most of us are in a position where there's room for improvement on both sides of the power-to-weight equation. We can get both stronger and lighter. This can happen simultaneously as you focus your training with the intervals starting on page 256 and the plans starting on page 243. But I caution you to resist going overboard on both at the same time. That is, don't train your brains out while slashing your food intake. That'll just make you slower, as a recent study of cyclists doing just that revealed.

For 10 weeks, researchers at Southern Connecticut State University in New Haven followed four groups of cyclists. One was told to integrate high-intensity interval sessions into their training while maintaining their weight. Another was told to continue their nor-

Pro Power

There's a reason those cyclists you see on your streaming race feed are paid to ride. They produce enough watts to light up a house. Here's a snapshot of average pro power.

TIME	PRO WOMEN	PRO MEN
10 seconds	900+ watts	1200+ watts
4 to 8 minutes	300–350 watts (5–5.5/kg)	425–450 watts (6–6.5/kg)
20 to 40 minutes	225–275 watts (4–4.5/kg)	350–375 watts (5–5.5/kg)
1 to 2 hours	175–225 watts (3.5–4/kg)	300–350 watts (4–5/kg)
2 to 4 hours	100–150 watts (1.5–2.5/kg)	200–250 watts (2–4/kg)

mal training while following a weight loss diet. A third was instructed to diet and add high-intensity interval work. And the fourth was told to just stay the course, continuing their normal training and eating.

How'd it work out? The interval-only group boosted their power-to-weight ratio by about 10 percent, despite no change in weight. Those who dieted also increased their power-to-weight ratio by an impressive margin—just over 9 percent—by shedding about 11 pounds, on average. Those who dieted and did interval training? No improvement. Zilch. None. Despite the fact that they dropped about 12 pounds. Instead of making them stronger, the weight loss weakened them, likely because they were underfueled for their workouts, or because they didn't have sufficient nutrients on board to build muscle, or both.

Your Rides in Watts

You've likely heard fellow riders chatting about how many watts they pulled on this ride or that. What does it mean? For those who don't track watts, here's a snapshot of average cycling watts at every riding intensity. *Note:* The wattage figures below are based on averages for fit, trained recreational cyclists.

RIDE TYPE	HEART RATE ZONE PERCEIVED AVERAGE WATTS (% MAX HEART RATE)	EXERTION (1–10)	AVERAGE CYCLING WATTS (MEN/WOMEN)*
Cruising the boardwalk	65–70	3–4	125/80
Brisk charity ride	70–85	5–6	175/120
Group hammerfest	85–90	7–8	200/150
Tossing-cookies hard	90+	9–10	250+/200+
10 seconds full throttle	100	10	500+/400+

*Based on 170 lb. man/125 lb. woman

That doesn't mean you can't clean up your eating while training hard. Let's face it, most of us could easily lose a few pounds by just being a little more careful about how many beers, nachos, or second servings we help ourselves to. But aggressively trying to lose weight while also training hard is counterproductive. If you're gung ho about weight loss, do it during the low-intensity parts of your training, like during the maintenance period, a good month or two before you start to build intensity for the season.

PART 3

FAST NUTRITION

Get a taste—literally—for speed!

Pasta Can Improve Your Riding.
—Bicycling magazine, January 2012

Last winter I was sitting in my office writing this very book you're holding in your hands when the January/February issue of *Bicycling* magazine hit my desk. On the cover in the bottom left-hand corner, right over "The Best New $2,000 Road Bikes," was the eye-catching line above. *Confession:* I shook my head and laughed out loud.

Not because it isn't true. It is. Rather, I was laughing because sports nutrition has become so convoluted over the years that simple tried-and-true prerace rituals like the spaghetti dinner have been crucified so thoroughly that "pasta can improve your riding" is actually news we can boldly proclaim in 2012. Plus, I should add . . . the story inside the magazine was mine. *I* proclaimed it. While I'm in confessional mode, I should also own up to being part of the original problem. Heck, just the previous year, I myself had written a feature for *Bicycling* titled "Big Fat Lies," in which I semi-bashed the popularly celebrated "pasta party." (Though, to be fair, I did say that pasta before a big ride is still a good thing.)

So what's the truth? Well, that's the thing. It's all true. Pasta *can* make you fast. Pasta can also make you fat. It depends on how much you eat, when you eat it, the type of riding or racing you're doing, and even your own personal metabolism. With all these variables, is it any wonder we're all (including the scientists themselves) so confused about the role pasta and other starchy carbs play in a cyclist's diet?

CUTTING THROUGH THE CLUTTER

My goal in this section is to talk about nutrition through the prism of cycling performance. What you want to eat to get fast and be fast. Though you'll find advice on what to eat, when to eat it, and how to lose weight, this is not a diet book. This is a sports performance book. I'm assuming that you're active. So the food advice within these pages is different from what I would write if I was dishing out advice for someone in the general population who might take a walk every now and then.

In the chapters that follow, you'll find the latest in sports nutrition research, particularly regarding carbs (because there's utter mass confusion out there, especially now that gluten is public enemy number one), protein (ditto in the confusion department), and fat (double ditto). I'll be completely up front and I will do my very best to cut through the clutter.

Sports nutrition science is ever evolving and by no means cut-and-dried. Over the past year alone, I've had my head spun around and sideways by two very accomplished, respected scientists. One believes you can't get the carbs (or the hydration) you need through sports drinks and that you should eat your food and drink your water, albeit with some electrolytes. The other is adamant that you never have to chew real food if you have the right beverage. I actually think they're both right. Again, it just depends. You'll find suggestions on how to perform your own trial and error to find what is right for you.

When it comes to using fuel to go fast, what you eat is only half the equation (and maybe not even the most essential half). Timing your nutrition is essential. When you put fuel in your tank determines how well you power off the line and—most important—whether or not you can keep the power up all the way to the finish, whether you're doing a 40-minute cross race or a 150-K gran fondo.

There's also the little matter of electrolytes. The most cutting-edge research says bonking, what we've known for decades to be glycogen depletion, might not be the product of an empty tank after all, but rather depleted spark plugs (i.e., electrolytes), so you're left with no ignition and unable to turn the stores you have into energy.

We'll talk sports supplements as well. Sadly, there are no pills that can transform you from a Cat 3 to a Tour contender, but there are a few supplements that can do just as the name implies—supplement your training to improve your results and, yes, make you faster.

Finally, if you're one of the roughly 220 million Americans who want to lose a little weight, you'll get the lowdown on how to determine how much energy you burn just sitting around (i.e., your resting metabolism) as well as how much you burn on your bike and how much you should eat to tip the scales, literally, in your favor. Grab your fork and let's dig in.

8

Fast Fuel

How much do you need to be fast?

> Cyclists eat too much.
> —Eddy Merckx

Last year, I was standing in a crowded venue in Manhattan, rapt along with dozens of other cycling enthusiasts, listening to Eddy Merckx spin tales about the glory days and what he did differently, what made him, well, Eddy Merckx. We all knew that he "rode lots" and had a passion that eclipsed his competition. But he made one simple statement that sent little murmured shock waves through the crowd: "Cyclists eat too much." In his hunger to go faster than the rest, Eddy let himself be a little hungry.

How much we need to eat is a question that has bedeviled cyclists for decades and continues to do so today. We've all heard the tales of pros meticulously weighing every morsel they put in their mouths. It stands in stark contrast to the notion that you should stuff yourself like a Christmas goose if you're racing the next day. Which way is right? It depends on your riding, your metabolism, and your goals.

On a day-to-day basis, we cyclists really do need less food than we think. Why? Because we're generally fuel efficient. We have speedy hybrid engines that can churn down the road for miles and miles without blowing through our stored fuel (glycogen). It's a product of training. (That's why new riders are more prone to bonking. They haven't laid the foundation to become fuel-efficient fat burners yet.) The more trained we become, the easier it is for us to bang out 30 or 40 miles, burning fewer calories as we do so (unless we're pushing it) because we're just not working as hard. So we can eat less to do the same work. Eddy didn't need exercise scientists to tell him that. He just knew.

Does that mean you have to parcel out your meager food portions like a pauper if you want to be fast? Heck no. You're still burning more calories than the average person. Your cycling life still allows you leeway to enjoy ample amounts of food. It's a matter of reeling back the excesses, passing up that third slice of tomato pie (and maybe the third brew) that you'd normally justify because, "Hey, I rode two hours today."

For most of us, it's also a matter of retraining our brains to know how much food is satisfying, rather than automatically dumping 4 cups of pasta on our plates because that's what the chain Italian restaurants do. In our calorie-polluted environment, we've all become victims of portion distortion. So it's going to take a little practice (and a few tricks) to dial in the right diet for riding fast. But I promise it'll be more sporting than spartan.

Note that this chapter deals solely with what you should be eating on a daily basis when you're in regular riding mode. Races and training days will be addressed in Chapter 9.

THE CALORIE EQUATION

A few months ago I spent a splendid sunny Saturday sitting in a conference room in a hotel off Times Square in New York City, racking up some continuing education credits at the annual Town Sports

International Summit and Trade Show. My last session for the day was "Turbo Fuel," led by Dominique Adair, MS, RD. The session promised to bring me up-to-date on the latest in nutrient timing, supplements, bars, and sports drinks.

In walked a whippet of a woman, blonde, lean, and petite with delicate bone structure and sinewy muscles. She introduced herself

Dominique Sample Day

Breakfast

1 bowl oatmeal with raisins & skim milk

1 banana

4 scrambled egg whites

1 cup coffee with whole milk

Snack

medium apple with 2 Tbsp peanut butter

Lunch

1 can tuna with 2 tsp soy mayo

large bowl raw spinach

1 whole wheat pita

1 cup chocolate soy milk

Snack

2 oz low-fat cheese

10 baby carrots

Dinner

Bowl of whole wheat pasta with 4 oz ground turkey, red sauce & broccoli

Large bowl mixed lettuce with 2 tsp vinaigrette

1 cup fresh orange juice

1 cup low-fat frozen yogurt

and told us she was a runner. Then she flashed a page from one of her daily diet logs on the overhead screen.

She turned to us and asked, "How many calories a day do you think that is?"

We started calling out numbers—1,600, 2,000, 1,800, and so forth—as she stood there silently smiling. The actual amount: 2,753. See the breakdown below.

"Wow," I thought. "That's not a ton of food and it's a fair amount

Food List Summary Report

FOOD ITEM	AMOUNT	WEIGHT (grams)	CALS	
Oatmeal	1.5 c	351	218	
Banana, Extra Large	1 ea	152	140	
Seedless Raisins	0.25 c	41	124	
Skim Milk	1 c	246	101	
Egg Whites	4 ea	134	67	
Whole Milk	0.25 T	61	37	
Apple, Large	1 oz	212	125	
Natural Peanut Butter	2 T	32	187	
Light Tuna	6 oz	170	197	
Soy Mayonnaise	2 t	28	198	
Spinach, Raw	2 c	60	13	
Soy Milk	1 c	245	81	
Whole Wheat Pita	1 ea	64	170	
Low-fat Cheese	2 oz	57	98	
Baby Carrots-Raw	10 ea	100	38	
Small Shell Pasta	2 c	230	324	
Lean Ground Turkey	4 oz	113	169	
Marinara Sauce	0.5 c	125	71	
Broccoli Spear	2 ea	62	17	
Fresh Orange Juice	1 c	248	112	
Low-fat Frozen Yogurt	1 c	193	219	
Oil & Vinegar	2 t	10	47	
	Totals	**2934**	**2753**	

of calories. So cyclists probably do eat too much; but they still need to eat an awful lot to maintain a lean, fast frame." How much? Let's take a look.

The amount of energy (i.e., calories) each of us needs is determined by our energy output—how many calories we expend living, breathing, riding our bikes, and so forth. Not surprisingly, the bulk of the calories you burn go to what's known as *basal metabolism,* the act of simply existing. The other major energy burners are physical

PROT (g)	CARB (g)	FIBER (g)	FAT (g)	SAT (g)	CHOL (mg)	SOD (mg)
9	38	6	4	1	0	4
2	36	4	1	0	0	2
1	33	2	0	0	0	5
10	14	0	1	0	5	145
14	1	0	0	0	0	219
2	3	0	2	1	8	30
0	32	6	1	0	0	0
8	7	2	16	2	0	80
43	0	0	1	0	51	575
0	1	0	22	3	16	157
2	2	2	0	0	0	47
7	4	3	5	1	0	29
6	35	5	2	0	0	340
14	1	0	4	2	12	347
1	8	2	1	0	0	35
11	65	3	2	0	0	2
20	0	0	9	3	90	107
2	10	2	3	0	0	515
2	3	2	0	0	0	17
2	26	0	0	0	0	2
10	42	3	4	2	10	113
0	0	0	5	1	0	0
165	**361**	**41**	**81**	**19**	**192**	**2771**

activity—everything from fidgeting to Spinning to eating, as it takes a good bit of energy to digest and break down the food you take in.

Here's a snapshot of how your metabolism is broken down by percentage.

BASAL METABOLISM: 60% to 75%

THERMIC EFFECT OF ACTIVITY: 15% to 30%

THERMIC EFFECT OF FOOD: 10%

In this case, a person eating 2,000 calories a day would burn approximately 1,400 to keep their organs functioning, 400 for activity, and 200 for digestion. The "thermic effect of activity" percentages displayed above are for relatively inactive people. Cyclists can expect to require 75 percent (or even pushing 100 percent) above basal metabolism to keep their working muscles fueled and in optimal working order.

Your basal metabolism is determined by myriad factors, including:

BODY COMPOSITION: While the number of calories muscle burns has been grossly exaggerated in the media, it still is a significant part of your furnace, as muscle burns three to five times more calories than fat does.

AGE: Your metabolism is highest when you're a growing teen. As you approach 40 and beyond, it slides back to the tune of about 2 to 5 percent per decade, largely due to muscle loss and fat gain.

GENDER: Women are generally smaller and have proportionally more fat and less muscle. Therefore our basal metabolic rate (BMR) is around 5 to 10 percent lower.

SIZE: The bigger you are, the more calories you burn. That's why dropping those last 5 pounds can feel impossible, because your body has reset its thermostat.

HORMONES: Your thyroid is the primary regulator of the hormones that govern metabolic rate.

The most accurate way to calculate your basal metabolism is to go to a lab where scientists use a gas-analysis machine to measure your oxygen consumption. It's easier to use some formulas, such as the Mifflin-St. Jeor equation below, though. The Mifflin-St. Jeor equation is what medical nutrition clinics use to determine the calorie requirements of patients, and research pitting it against gas analysis shows the formula generally produces accurate results. It looks a little intimidating at first glance, but once you pop in your weight (in kilograms; one kilogram equals 2.2 pounds) and height (in centimeters; one centimeter equals 2.54 inches), it's not that hard to work through.

Calculate Your BMR

MALE	10×weight ✚ 6.25×height ✚ 5×age ✚ 5 ≡ BMR
FEMALE	10×weight ✚ 6.25×height ✚ 5×age ━ 161 ≡ BMR

Now add in your activity level. Multiply your BMR by the following, depending on how much riding and other activities you do.

1.200	≡	sedentary (little or no exercise)
1.375	≡	lightly active (light exercise/sports 1–3 days/week, approx. 590 Cal/day)
1.550	≡	moderately active (moderate exercise/sports 3–5 days/week, approx. 870 Cal/day)
1.725	≡	very active (hard exercise/sports 6–7 days a week, approx. 1150 Cal/day)
1.900	≡	extra active (very hard exercise/sports and physical job, approx. 1580 Cal/day)

The number you end up with is the number of calories you should be eating every day to maintain your weight and fuel your riding. Obviously, if you want to lose weight, you need to take in fewer calories than you're burning, to the tune of about 250 to 500 fewer a day. I would never advocate spending the rest of your life counting calories, but I do believe that a few days of tallying can be eye-opening and give you a working idea of how 2,500 or 3,000 or whatever number of calories you need each day physically looks and feels.

There are a number of great calorie-counting apps available for your tablet or smartphone that make tallying your intake pretty easy. You'll find a rundown of the best online calorie counters as well as other weight loss advice in Chapter 10. For now, let's concentrate on where the calories you eat should be coming from.

THE RIGHT "MACRO MIX" TO RIDE FAST

Carbohydrates, protein, and fat. Those are the three macronutrients everyone needs to live. As cyclists, we need them to fuel our riding, repair our muscles, and keep our energy systems firing on all cylinders. Forget everything you've heard over the past two decades about fat being evil. Oh, no, it's carbs that are evil. Or maybe it's just certain fats and carbs that are evil . . . or maybe not so much.

In the quest to find the devil behind our country's obesity crisis, diet "gurus" have demonized one or more of these essential macronutrients, only to end up with everyone getting fatter anyway. Ignore the hype and tune in to the hard facts. As a cyclist, you need a balance of all three macronutrients to ride—especially if you want to ride fast.

What's the right mix? It depends who you ask. Traditionalists will tell you endurance athletes like cyclists should aim for 60 percent carbs, 20 percent protein, and 20 percent fat. Others go for a more even 40 percent carbs, 30 percent protein, 30 percent fat approach. Both are fairly good breakdowns, but I've never been very convinced they're that useful. What does 20 percent fat look like? It's not like you're going to plop a serving of lard on your plate next to your pile of rice, green salad, and hunk of chicken. So while it helps to know that you should be getting over half (sometimes considerably more) of your calories from carbs and about a quarter each from protein and fat, it's far better to know how much of each you should actually be eating.

It's also important to address where these macronutrients come from. You could conceivably hit all the right ratios with a bowl of popcorn, a hot dog, and a milk shake, but that won't get you very far. By eating the right amount of the highest-quality macronutrients, you'll fuel, restock, and repair your muscles to keep riding strong through all your training cycles.

CARBOHYDRATES: YOUR FASTEST FUEL

Your body doesn't use carbohydrates as building blocks. They are fuel, period. So to use the tried-and-true car analogy, how much you need depends on how far and/or how fast you're going. Just as you wouldn't go out and pour more gas into your parked car if you weren't going anywhere, you don't need to be topping off your own fuel stores when you're not riding much and don't plan to any time soon. Conversely, if you're riding 200 miles a week, you need to keep that tank full so you don't hit empty.

Stacy Sims, PhD, is a Stanford-based exercise physiologist and nutrition scientist who has consulted for pro teams and runs Osmo Nutrition. She recommends the following guidelines for matching your overall daily carb intake to how much activity you do. Each gram of carbohydrate provides four calories of energy.

EXERCISE LEVEL	RECOMMENDED DAILY CARBOHYDRATE*
Low/Easy: <1 hour of training per day	205 to 275 grams
Moderate: About an hour of training per day	275 to 340 grams
Very Active: 1 to 3 hours of training per day	410 to 475 grams
Extremely Active: 4 to 5 hours or more of training per day	545 to 580 grams

*For a 150 lb. cyclist

As you'll see in the Chapter 9, which covers nutrient timing and carbo-loading, it's especially important to hit those higher marks before a hard race or century ride, particularly if you're going for speed. A study published in the *International Journal of Sports Medicine* reported that endurance athletes who consumed more than 7 grams of carbs per kilogram of body weight (that works out to about 475 grams for a 150-pound rider) the day before a race posted significantly faster times and maintained speed better than those who ate fewer than that amount.

Now comes the more confusing part: Where should these carbs be coming from? Most of use *starch* and *carb* almost interchangeably. While spaghetti and bagels are indeed carbohydrates, and you do need carbohydrates for fuel, starch is not the only source, nor is it always the best source, especially if you're trying to stay at fighting (or climbing) weight. Starchy carbs turn to sugar quickly—one analogy I've always loved is that spaghetti is just sugar on a string—and are as easy to overeat as potato chips, because your brain operates on sugar. When it gets a rush from a bagel or a piece of cake, it leaves you wanting more, so you eat more than you need, which of course gets stocked away in your fat stores. A starch-based diet also makes your body become more of a sugar (rather than fat) burner, so you bonk more easily as well as eat too much. It also explains why you may get an energy crash 30 to 45 minutes after your morning bagel.

Fruits and vegetables, on the other hand, are rich in carbohydrates, but tend to be lower in calories and slower to digest. You're also pretty unlikely to go on a broccoli binge, and it would be less damaging to your diet if you did. As a big bonus, plant foods are loaded with vitamins, minerals, and immunity-boosting phytonutrients that make you healthier and stronger, so you can ride better and burn more calories.

I used the following approach myself with much success. When I first started riding, I was a bit of a starch hound. To me, if it didn't end with an *i* (*rotini, ziti, fusilli*), it wasn't fuel. I had never stopped to think that carbs come in many shapes and sizes, or that as a cyclist, I actually burned a lot of fat for fuel. Then I started doing some searching around. I read about how Allen Lim, PhD, coauthor of the *The Feed Zone Cookbook* and a brilliant mind in cycling science, had eliminated wheat from his Tour riders' diets and was feeding them rice cakes filled with eggs, olive oil, prosciutto, and liquid amino acids. Even Joe Friel, who was a carbo-loading king in his Training Bible series, was promoting a low-starch Paleo-based diet of vegetables, fruits, and lean meats as fuel.

With nothing to lose but a few extra pounds that seemed stuck on my frame, I overhauled my eating. I limited starches to a small quarter-portion on my plate and piled on broccoli, brussels sprouts, leafy greens, nuts, fruits, and lean meats. Within a couple of months, I went from weighing 130-something to weighing 120-something. And there I have stayed, nearly effortlessly. The best part: I rarely even come close to bonking, and I feel like I can ride much longer and faster on far less food.

A bonus of following this Paleo-like diet is that when you do eat starch (and there are times you need it), it's like high-octane fuel.

Gluten Confusion

Will going gluten free make you faster? A lot of racers seem to think so, as evidenced by the likes of Christian Vande Velde and Tom Danielson attributing their newfound energy, recovery, and improved sleep to gluten-free diets (as recommended to them by Allen Lim, PhD, coauthor of the The Feed Zone Cookbook).

Gluten is a protein found in wheat grain. About 1 in 133 people—or 1.5 million Americans—are officially gluten intolerant, a condition known as celiac disease. In other words, they can't digest the stuff, which can cause a host of gastrointestinal woes as well as fatigue. Another untold number of people have wheat allergies that cause rashes, breathing problems, and nausea. Some experts also claim that even more people have nonceliac gluten intolerance, meaning that they'll test negative for celiac disease (which is screened through a blood test), but still don't digest gluten optimally. The only way to know if you have nonceliac intolerance is to pull gluten from your diet and see how you feel.

Finding gluten-free foods is pretty easy now that going gluten free is so popular. In general, you'd be swapping your wheat-based pasta and bread for rice, oats, corn, quinoa, and other food made from those gluten-free sources. Will going gluten free transform your cycling? The dietitians I consulted, including Stacy Sims, PhD, of Stanford University, weren't convinced it would unless you had discernible symptoms of gluten intolerance. But you may lose some weight and feel better if going gluten free means cutting out sweets, refined starches, and beer.

Case in point: I was racing the Breck Epic last summer. It's a 6-day, 240-mile race based out of Breckenridge, Colorado, that starts at around 9,000 feet of elevation and routinely climbs into five digits, including two trips over 12,000 feet of altitude. By week's end, you go up and down those mighty Rocky Mountains so many times you accumulate nearly 37,000 feet of vertical climbing. That whole week, I started the day with a big fat bagel and finished it up with a bed of rice (topped with everything) and a dinner roll as a chaser. I still ate plenty of fruits and vegetables and protein. But there's no question the starch helped stuff my glycogen stores and kept me going.

WHERE THE CARBS ARE

Here's a snapshot of how fruits and vegetables compare with pasta and other traditional starchy carb sources.

VEGETABLES (SERVING SIZE)	CARBS (GRAMS)
Artichokes, cooked (1 medium)	13 g
Beets, cooked (½ cup)	8 g
Broccoli, raw (1 cup)	4 g
Brussels sprouts, cooked (½ cup)	7 g
Cabbage, cooked (½ cup)	3 g
Carrots, cooked (½ cup)	8 g
Cauliflower, cooked (½ cup)	3 g
Celery, raw (1 cup)	4 g
Collard greens, cooked (1 cup)	12 g
Corn, sweet, cooked (1oz)	7 g
Eggplant, cooked (1 cup)	7 g
Kale, cooked (1 cup)	7 g
Leeks, cooked (½ cup)	4 g
Mushrooms, raw (1 cup)	4 g
Onions, raw (1 cup)	14 g
Parsnips, cooked (½ cup)	15 g
Peas, green, cooked (1 cup)	25 g
Peppers, green (1 cup)	10 g
Pumpkin, cooked, mashed (1 cup)	12 g
Radishes, raw (1 cup)	4 g

VEGETABLES (SERVING SIZE)	CARBS (GRAMS)
Spinach, cooked (1 cup)	7 g
Squash, winter, acorn, cooked (1 cup)	30 g
Succotash, cooked (1 cup)	47 g
Sweet potato, baked w/skin (large)	44 g
Swiss chard, cooked (1 cup)	7 g
Tomatoes, raw (1 cup)	8 g
Turnips, cooked, mashed (1 cup)	11 g
Zucchini, cooked (1 cup)	8 g

FRUIT (SERVING SIZE)	CARBS (GRAMS)
Bananas (1 medium)	30 g
Cantaloupe (1 cup)	15 g
Grapes (1 cup)	16 g
Kiwi fruit (1 large)	14 g
Honeydew (1 cup)	16 g
Mangoes (1 regular)	35 g
Nectarines (1 medium)	16 g
Oranges (1 medium)	14 g
Peaches (1 large)	17 g
Pears (1 medium)	25 g
Pineapple (1 cup)	19 g
Plums (1 medium)	8 g
Pomegranates, raw (1 medium)	26 g
Raisins, seedless (¼ cup)	32 g
Raspberries (1 cup)	14 g
Strawberries (1 cup)	11 g
Tangerines, mandarin oranges (1 medium)	8 g
Watermelon (1 cup)	11 g

PASTA AND GRAINS	CARBS (GRAMS)
French bread (5")	18 g
Italian bread (1 large slice)	15 g
Long grain rice, brown (1 cup)	45 g
Long grain rice, white (1 cup)	45 g
Macaroni (1 cup)	40 g
Macaroni, whole wheat (1 cup)	37 g
Mixed grain bread (1 large slice)	15 g
Oatmeal (1 cup)	22 g
Pita bread, white (6" diameter)	33 g
Pita bread, whole wheat (6" diameter)	35 g
Pumpernickel bread (1 slice)	12 g
Rye bread (1 slice)	15 g
Short grain rice, white (1 cup)	37 g
Sourdough bread (1 large slice)	18 g
Spaghetti (1 cup)	40 g
Spaghetti, whole wheat (1 cup)	37 g
Tagliatelle (1 cup)	44 g
Wheat bread (1 slice)	12 g

PROTEIN: BUILT FOR SPEED

Unlike carbohydrates, protein isn't a primary fuel source. Rather, it is an essential structural building block that is best known for building muscle. It's also a major player in immunity, hormone and enzyme regulation, sleep, and digestion. Though you don't burn much protein for fuel, your protein needs still vary according to your training volume and intensity. Not surprisingly, the more you ride and train, the more protein you need.

To figure out your daily protein quota, calculate between 0.5 and 0.8 grams of protein per pound of body weight, or between 75 and 120 grams a day for a 150-pound rider. You'll want to skew on the higher end when you're in a particularly hard training block. In fact, you should even push that a little higher if you're deep in training and racing stress. In a study recently published in *Medicine and Science in Sports and Exercise,* researchers found that cyclists pushing all the way to 3 grams of protein per kilogram of body weight (so, 200 grams for a 150-pound rider) recovered better and felt less stressed during high-intensity training blocks than those eating lesser amounts.

That's because amino acids repair your hardworking muscles and help them come back stronger. Your body also dips into your protein stores as you ride, especially if your glycogen supply runs low. About 3 to 8 percent of your riding energy needs are supplied by branched-chain amino acids (BCAAs), specifically leucine, isoleucine, and valine, which are found in many protein-rich foods. Without enough of these BCAAs for your muscles to oxidize for energy, your performance declines and riding feels harder.

I'm a huge proponent of eating your protein early to front-load your day, mostly because it promotes satiety and helps provide more even energy, so you'll be less likely to overeat later. After talking with protein researcher Donald Layman, PhD, of the University of Illinois in Urbana, I became even further convinced. He explained that you start the day in a catabolic (muscle-devouring) state following your overnight fast. Most people get a measly 10 grams of protein from their morning meal, which isn't nearly enough to fully restock your stores and does little to regulate your appetite for the day ahead. To meet those needs, Layman advises aiming for 30 grams of protein at breakfast to stimulate muscle growth and blunt your appetite. That's two eggs and a Greek yogurt.

As you may have heard, there are complete and incomplete

sources of protein. Put simply, protein comes in two varieties, complete and incomplete. Complete protein sources are those that contain all nine amino acids. You can find complete proteins in meat, fish, eggs, most dairy products, and soybean foods such as tofu. Plant sources, such as nuts, whole grains, and vegetables, are usually incomplete sources, meaning they're missing some amino acids. The good news is that foods we naturally eat in concert, such as beans and rice and peanut butter on bread work together to make a complete protein. There's no need to stress about combining foods to make a complete protein at every meal. As long as you take in all the amino acids you need within a day, you'll get all the complete protein you need.

The easiest way to get more protein is to change the composition of your plate, making sure there's a nice one-quarter to one-third portion devoted to protein. Also, load up on vegetables, which contribute to your overall protein number at a very low calorie cost. Here's a look at some high-quality protein sources that add up.

FOOD	PROTEIN (GRAMS)
Steak (4 oz)	34 g
Chicken breast (4 oz)	26 g
Pork (4 oz)	26 g
Tuna (4 oz)	26 g
Salmon (3 oz)	19 g
Greek yogurt (6 oz)	18 g
Shrimp (3 oz)	18 g
Whitefish (3 oz)	16 g
Yogurt, low-fat plain (1 cup)	13 g
Eggs (2)	12 g
Tofu (4 oz)	11 g

FOOD	PROTEIN (GRAMS)
Lentils (½ cup)	9 g
Peanut butter (2 Tbsp)	8 g
Cheese (1 oz/1 slice)	7 g
Nuts (1 oz)	7 g
Pasta (1 cup)	7 g
Mixed vegetables (⅔ cup)	2 g

FAT: A SPEED "DEMON"

Remember that part about your being a hybrid engine? That means you need to be eating fat. Fat is not evil. Fat is good. Fat is healthy. Fat is fuel. You need fat to repair cell membranes, maintain healthy immunity, and optimize your hormone levels. Fat does not make you fat. The word has gotten such negative connotations, I almost feel like we need to start calling it something else. But in the meantime, believe this, eating enough fat will help make you fast.

How much is enough? Forget the standard 20-percent-of-your-calories-from-fat rule. That should be a minimum. Research shows that athletes who eat diets higher in fat, around 30+ percent (that's about 70 grams in a 2,000-calorie-per-day diet), produce better average times to exhaustion in exercise tests than those eating your typical low-fat, high-carb diet.

Again, the fitter you are, the better a fat burner you become. So if long rides are part of your usual repertoire, you can push your fat intake up to 35 or even 40 percent for performance benefits. The easiest way for most cyclists to get the fat they need is simply to not intentionally avoid it, since it's naturally found in so many foods we eat daily.

That's not to say you should go whole hog with the burgers, fries, and ribs, of course. Though even saturated fat isn't the nutritional bogeyman it once was, there are far healthier types of fat, particularly monounsaturated and polyunsaturated fats, which you're very likely not getting enough of. Experts recommend getting about 20 percent of your fat from these healthy types of fat. Good sources for those include fatty fish such as salmon, tuna, and mackerel, as well as avocado, nuts, plant oils, olives, and even grass-fed beef.

Interestingly, in an interview with the blog Belgium Knee Warmers, pro cycling team manager Jonathan Vaughters detailed how, after discovering that Tour contender Tom Danielson was a

Fishing for Omega-3s

Omega-3s are instrumental in nearly every function of your body, from generating healthy cells to forming the building blocks of your brain and eyes. They turn genes on and off, help cells communicate with one another, fight infection, and maybe most important, quell inflammation, which is very important for active cyclists. Unfortunately, these essential fatty acids are not so easy to come by. They're found in small doses in nuts and some plants, but the best source for complete omega-3 fatty acids is fish, especially cold water varieties such as mackerel, sardines, and wild salmon. Aim to take in about 1,000 milligrams a day. The easiest way, as you can see, is by eating fish a few times a week.

FOOD	OMEGA-3 (MILLIGRAMS)
Mackerel (3½ oz)	2,600 mg
Salmon (3½ oz)	1,500 mg
Anchovies (3½ oz)	1,400 mg
Tuna (6 oz albacore)	1,280 mg
Beef, lean (3 oz, grass fed)	136 mg
Eggs (omega-3 fortified, 2)	114 mg

terrible fat burner, nearly burning sugar exclusively and cracking on long rides as a result, the team completely changed his diet, moving him away from standard carbs and filling him up with nuts, protein, and guacamole. After two months, Danielson was cranking out 6-hour rides without even finishing the energy bars in his pockets.

I'm no Tour rider, but I found the exact same thing happened when I made the switch. I needed far less food on 4-, even 5-hour mountain bike rides, and I rarely ever hit the wall.

ELECTROLYTES: TO KEEP FIRING FAST

Here's an interesting fact: Though most of us think of bonking as a state of glycogen depletion—our fuel tank hitting empty—scientists have gone to great lengths to prove otherwise. Case in point: Esteemed sports researchers Timothy Noakes, MD, and Dan Benardot, PhD, RD, LD, have conducted studies where they had athletes exercise until they hit the wall to complete exhaustion only to find they had plenty of glycogen still on board.

In one such study, they worked a group of athletes to fatigue, then numbed their central nervous systems and artificially stimulated their muscles. Their muscles continued to fire, which if they were out of glycogen, they wouldn't have been able to do. In another study, they drove the athletes to exhaustion with a 4-hour exercise test, while continually testing their muscle glycogen concentrations and carbohydrate-burning rates. Guess what? Those levels and rates were the same when they were staggeringly exhausted at 4 hours as they had been an hour previous at the 3-hour mark. They still had gas, but zero go.

What's going on? Scientists are still working on that. But suffice it to say, bonking is a bit more complicated than we once thought. Your brain ultimately governs your muscles and it takes care of them by continuously monitoring core temperature, blood volume, sweat rate, fuel stores, and stress hormones. If it doesn't like what it sees, it pulls the plug to protect you—glycogen stores be damned.

One surefire way to keep your muscles firing quickly and smoothly longer is to keep your electrolytes balanced, something too many of us overlook. Electrolytes are charged salts and minerals, specifically sodium, potassium, calcium, and magnesium, that help create the electrical impulses that transmit messages from your brain to your muscles. They also serve as conductors for the cells, allowing fluids and nutrients and waste to be carried to all the right places. That means they help keep you hydrated, which in turn helps control core body temperature and neutralize lactic acid and other metabolic waste acids that are dumped into the bloodstream by your working muscles.

Some of the brightest minds in sports medicine today, such as Drs. Lim and Sims, believe that most late-event performance drops or blowups aren't related to nutrition at all, but rather electrolyte depletion. That's because even if you have enough fuel on board, without your spark plugs, you have no ignition and are left powerless. This "electrolyte bonk" can leave you cramped, weak, headachy, and nauseous.

As you probably know, sodium is the electrolyte you lose in the greatest amounts through sweat, as you shed about 300 to 700 milligrams per hour depending on your sweat rate. So it's also the electrolyte you need to replace most. Sports nutritionists generally recommend replacing your sodium at a rate of 250 to 500 milligrams an hour. For the best results, look for a product that provides the full spectrum of electrolytes, as well as some B vitamins (which help the body convert stored fuel into energy), and maybe a little caffeine (which frees fatty acids, stimulates the central nervous system, and helps lower perceived exertion during exercise)—all of which keep you going faster longer.

In a study of 14 cyclists who pedaled for 2 hours and then completed a 15-minute performance test, those who drank an electrolyte sports drink spiked with B vitamins, caffeine, and some amino acids performed better, maintained better leg strength, and reported feeling lower rates of perceived exertion (the work felt easier) than those who drank an electrolyte sports drink without the additives.

There are many good electrolyte products on the market. Two favorites: Nuun and Zym sports drink tablets. They're portable, taste good, and provide the electrolytes and key vitamins you need without all the sugar you don't. Sims and others believe that drinking fluids that contain too many carbohydrates (sugars) slows absorption because your stomach has trouble sorting the sugars from the water. (As opposed to when you eat food separately, where it naturally forms a bolus in the gut.) So you have fluids sloshing in your gut and nothing is getting where it needs to be. If you've ever experienced that "gut rot" feeling from too much sports drink, you may have experienced this upset, bloated, irritable stomach sensation.

For longer rides—say more than 2½ hours—adding a little bit of sugar to the sodium electrolyte mix—say about 75 calories' worth per bottle—helps with absorption and stabilizes blood sugar as well. The new generation of sports drinks such as Osmo and Skratch Labs deliver about 80 calories per bottle as well as ample amounts of sodium (about two to three times what other energy drinks use), along with a dash of potassium and calcium. They also contain no artificial colors, flavors, or anything else. This may sound like an advertisement for the mixes, but it is actually pretty important for keeping up your speed. In Sim's work, she's found that artificial ingredients, especially sweeteners, can irritate the stomach (thus slowing nutrient absorption) and even have a laxative effect (that'll slow you down in a hurry) when taken during exertion.

HYDRATION: DRINK UP TO THROW DOWN

A few months ago, I was flipping through one of the many sports journals that regularly come across my desk when I stumbled upon a published study that I was a participant in. It was from the 2008 Ironman Louisville (the study itself spanned 2008 through 2010 races). Before we could pick up our registration packets, the volunteers asked us to step on a scale to check our hydration status. I confess to being less than thrilled—having been tapering and carbo-loading, I felt like a bloated tick and the last thing I needed before the 140-mile odyssey was to see a high number on the scale. But I obliged. The volunteer cheerfully informed me that at 64 percent (55 to 65 percent is considered adequate hydration), I was properly hydrated and ready to go.

In fact I was *really* ready to go. I had a great race despite temperatures that rose into the 90s Fahrenheit and went on to Kona six weeks later. Turns out maybe that hydration status really helped. The correlation between hydration status and finishing times was significant. The researchers reported that when all else was equal, for every 1 percent increase in hydration, the men's finish times decreased by 16 minutes and the women's by 12 minutes—they got that much faster. Among the men finishing in under 12 hours, the hydration levels were 68 percent or greater. Among the fastest women, the hydration levels were 63 percent or greater.

By no means does this mean you should drown yourself in fluids before (or during) even the hardest, longest rides. The goal is to go in adequately hydrated and keep yourself there. For the most part, that means drinking according to thirst. Top off your tank with 16 ounces of an electrolyte sports drink an hour or two before you saddle up. That will give your body time to absorb what it needs and eliminate what it doesn't. Then take in about 6 to 8 ounces (two to three gulps) every 15 to 20 minutes while you ride, or about a bottle an hour. Your thirst is actually a pretty good guide.

9

Fast-Fuel Timing

When you eat may be more important than what you eat when you need some speed.

Fast Fact: The rider who feasts the most on the bike finishes first. A postevent survey found that cyclists consumed about 53 grams (212 calories) of carbohydrates per hour, Ironman triathletes took in 70 grams (280 calories), and marathoners took in 35 grams (140 calories). Those who consumed the highest amounts had the best finishing times.

I was talking to Anne Guzman, a sports nutrition consultant for the Peaks Coaching Group and former pro bike racer, about the biggest nutrition mistakes she sees cyclists make. I fully expected her to say the usual—skipping breakfast, eating junk, misjudging their portions—the stuff all nutritionists say. Instead, she paused and gave a more nuanced (and far more interesting) reply. "They don't separate training foods and riding foods," she said. In other words, the meals and snacks that you eat during your everyday life should be very different from those you eat right before or during a bike ride. Too often, she explained, they're all mixed up and it's to our detriment. "I see riders stopping on long rides to have a chicken sandwich because they say they need protein, and then they eat energy bars for snacks at their desks. I just sit and think, 'What's wrong with this picture?'"

There's an awful lot wrong with that picture, because when it comes to performing well and riding fast, nutrient timing is everything. We're not camels. We can store only limited amounts of sustenance before we need replenishment. What we eat to stock our stores before we ride, what we eat to top off our reserves when we're out there going full throttle, and what we eat when the ride is in the books determine how fast and far we can go. Here's how to get the timing right.

BEFORE YOU RIDE

Let's say you're packing up to go on a long road trip. What's on the top of your list? Fuel up the car. Now let's say you're just dashing down to the library to return a book and maybe stop at the grocery store for milk and eggs. Chances are you don't even check the tank. You just go. Riding is pretty similar.

We all have plenty of stored energy (i.e., fat stores) for a relatively short, easy ride. So unless you're starving and on fumes, you don't need any special fueling for a semicasual hour or so outing. But let's say that hour-long outing is an interval workout. By nature of the intensity, you'll be sucking glycogen from your limited stores quickly, so you'll want to top off the tank before you head out.

Ask yourself two questions when you're planning your preride fuel: How long? How hard? Your goal is to have enough energy to perform your best without being weighed down or left ravenous and thus highly susceptible to overeating when you're done. In general, you want to stick to simple foods that are filling but not too heavy. This is also when you want to go ahead and fork down those starchy carbs that you might be avoiding at other times of the day.

"This is where you draw the line between your daily nutrition, where maybe you're eating mostly protein-based foods and vegetables, and your performance foods, when you need those starchy carbohydrates and sugars," says Guzman. "Above all, *eat*. Too many riders still underfuel their rides with the hopes of losing weight. It always backfires," she says.

"If you're undereating, you're not performing well. You're also emptying your glycogen, so your body has to perform gluconeogenesis—digging into your protein and lean muscle stores to make energy. Now you're breaking down your lean body tissue, which is where your strength comes from. It does no good to be skinny if you're off the back. And chances are you won't get skinny, because you'll finish the ride starving and eat everything in sight," notes Guzman.

Not a pretty picture. So fuel early, fuel often, and fuel right. Use the following chart as your guide:

YOUR RIDE IS:	
Easy and short (45 to 90 minutes)	**EAT THIS:** If you've had a meal recently, you're fine. If it's been more than 3 hours since you've eaten, have a small snack like a banana or a couple of fig bars before you go.
	WHEN: If you're not going hard, you can scarf down the food as you're kitting up. Digestion won't be an issue.
Easy and long (2+ hours)	**EAT THIS:** You'll be burning mostly fat, but you still need energy on board for the long haul. You want foods that leave your stomach at different rates so you have some quick energy as well as some slower-digesting, lasting energy to fend off hunger and fatigue as you pass the 90-minute mark. Go with a cup of yogurt with granola or an English muffin with nut butter.
	WHEN: About ½ hour before you roll. But timing isn't critical since digestion won't be a problem because you're not going hard..

YOUR RIDE IS:	
Moderate to tempo and short (45 to 90 minutes with some climbs and/or harder efforts)	**EAT THIS:** As the ride intensity rises, so does your need for glycogen (carbs). It also gets harder to digest food because blood leaves your stomach to feed your working muscles. Choose easily digestible carbs (i.e., not too high in fiber) with a little protein. Good choices are a small turkey sandwich or a cup of cereal with low-fat milk and berries.
	WHEN: About 2 hours before you pedal. Everyone has different digestion tolerance levels. You want enough time to digest your food, but not so much that you're feeling hungry again before you start.
Moderate to tempo and long (2+ hours with some climbs and/or harder efforts)	**EAT THIS:** You'll be out there working for a pretty long time, so you want to start with a fairly full tank. Good choices are peanut butter and honey on a bagel or a bowl of oatmeal with raisins.
	WHEN: About 2 hours preride. Since you'll be going longer, you'll also be taking food with you.
Hard and short (45 to 90 minutes; cyclocross practice, track workout, intervals)	**EAT THIS:** You're going to suck your glycogen stores dry, so it's essential that they start on full so you don't hit the wall before you've finished your final effort. Digestion will also be pretty compromised, so you don't want to eat anything that'll come sailing back up. That means not too much fat, which really stalls stomach emptying. Go with pancakes or waffles with fruit and some nuts such as pecans. Or try rice or pasta (lightly dressed) with some sliced turkey.
	WHEN: About 2½ to 3 hours ahead of time. You want plenty of time for your food to digest. About 15 minutes before go time, top your tank with 100 calories of something simple: a few sports chews, half an energy bar, or fig bars and a few swallows of sports drink.
Hard and long (2+ hours, or an epic beatdown of any variety)	**EAT THIS:** You're going to need food—carbs and plenty of them. Start by eating 400 to 600 calories, about 60 percent of them coming from carbohydrates. Try a breakfast burrito with eggs and cooked veggies with some potatoes or a rice or pasta bowl with cooked veggies, some tofu, and light dressing.
	WHEN: About 3 to 4 hours preride. You'll be eating a substantial amount of food and you want plenty of time for your food to digest. About 30 minutes before go time, top your tank with 100 to 200 calories of something simple: a few sports chews, half an energy bar, or fig bars and a few swallows of sports drink.

FOOD FOR THE RIDE

Even the leanest, meanest cyclist has 40,000 calories worth of stored fat—roughly enough to ride for about 3 days straight. But here's the problem: Fat burns in a carbohydrate flame. So without enough carbohydrates on board, your cells can't fully break down fat in the energy cycle. And guess what? You have just 2,000 calories' worth of carbs stored as glycogen in your muscles and liver—enough to make it roughly 90 minutes to 2 hours at a good clip.

That's why you need to take in a steady stream of carbs for rides that last longer than your glycogen store limits. How many you need depends again on how hard and how long you're going to be out there. The goal is not to replace all the energy you're burning. That would be nearly impossible when you consider that even on a moderate ride you're churning through about 500 calories an hour (more if you're going hard). Instead, you want to top off your reserves so you have enough glycogen to burn for energy and to perform fat metabolism.

To do that, you should aim to put back about half the calories you're burning per hour. A good starting point is about 200 to 400 calories an hour, with 50 to 80 grams of those being calories from carbohydrates. Now here's the important part and the thing that most of us screw up: Start eating those carbs right away (about 30 minutes or so into the ride) rather than waiting till you're pushing empty, especially if you're riding anything harder than an easy endurance pace. This will make a huge difference in how well you can maintain a steady, hard effort.

Why do you need food when you're already fueled? Because the faster you ride when you start out, the higher the percentage of carbs you burn. Your body also burns more carbs right out of the gate when your glycogen stores are full to the brim. If you wait till 90 minutes or 2 hours in to take a bite of food, your supplies may already be dwindling, which forces you to slow down to an easier,

Avoid Gut Rot

The longer you're out there, the harder your gastrointestinal (GI) system has to work. For ultraendurance riders—think 100-mile mountain bike races or Ironman-level events—avoiding "gut rot" (the cramped, bloated, nauseated, and/or gassy feeling you get when your GI system cries uncle) becomes priority number one.

The easiest way to avoid gut rot, as mentioned previously, is to eat real food. Energy bars and blocks have their place in a rider's diet, but a steady stream of them for hours on end is simply too much of a burden on your belly. I've always figured it was just the concentrated sugar that left me fighting nausea during long endurance rides and races (after about 6 hours or so). But Dr. Allen Lim, coauthor of the excellent *Feed Zone Cookbook,* contends that artificial colors, flavors, and sweeteners are equally culpable and can cause flavor fatigue and an irritable stomach and GI tract.

Some of his favorite energy foods for rides and races are homemade sweet, salty, and savory treats such as small boiled potatoes drizzled with olive oil, salt, and parmesan cheese; sushi rice cakes with a little bacon; waffle sandwiches; and tortillas filled with almond butter and honey.

The best part about these foods is that they provide a real mental lift along with a steady flow of physical energy. Sinking your teeth into a delicious homemade snack at mile 80-something feels like a treat; like you're nourishing yourself. Choking down some rock-hard energy bar, on the other hand, can be salt in your mental wounds when you're already feeling worked from the ride.

more fat-burning pace or risk hitting the wall. By eating something every 30 minutes, you can start fast and stay fast (we'll talk about how much you should be drinking in the next section).

Though there's a ceiling to how many carbs your body can absorb per minute (scientists used to think it was just 1 gram per minute; we now know it's quite a bit higher), the more you can tolerate, the better you'll do. The key is feeding your body from a variety of carb sources. There are different types of simple sugars such as glucose, fructose, and sucrose. You have individual transporters in your gut that break down each type and shuttle it into your bloodstream. But they can absorb only a fixed amount in any given time period. So if your glucose transporters are maxed out at 60 grams, others, like those for fructose, are still available.

In his lab, Asker Jeukendrup, PhD, the global senior director of the Gatorade Sports Science Institute in Barrington, Illinois, found that by using a drink blend that included fructose, he could get athletes to absorb a whopping 1.75 grams per minute—more than 100 grams or 400 calories an hour.

But you have to train your gut to handle that amount of fuel. That's right, *train your gut,* and it's something far too many riders neglect, according to experts like Jeukendrup. "Your gut is every bit as trainable, if not more trainable, than your legs. And every bit as important," he told me as we were chatting about what separates endurance champions from the rest of us. "If you only eat two hundred or two hundred fifty calories an hour in training, your gut won't suddenly accept twice that much during a race," he said. You need to gradually increase your carb intake during training to hit those high amounts.

As your gut becomes better at tolerating and absorbing calories during activity, your performance can improve exponentially. Even if you don't hit 400 calories an hour, if you keep a steady stream coming in (again, not dumping the whole load into your system at once), chances are you can absorb more than you imagine—and keep a faster, steadier pace as well.

Experiment with foods that you like and can tolerate. The sports nutrition market is saturated with energy bars of every variety, but real food works just as well, if not better. If you're heading out for a long ride of 3 or more hours, it's even more important to pack real food. In fact, it's usually better to start with real food such as peanut

Kick It Up a Notch with Caffeine

These days everything from gels to lip balm comes caffeinated. If you can tolerate it, by all means include caffeine in your cycling nutrition. Contrary to the old myths about this central nervous system stimulant, it does not have diuretic effects when you use it during exercise, so you won't pee more and get dehydrated. And it can most definitely improve your performance.

Numerous studies have shown that caffeine lowers your rate of perceived exertion while improving your strength, endurance, and mental performance. Even better, researchers from the University of Birmingham in England found that riders who drank a caffeinated sports beverage boosted their carb-burning rate by 26 percent over those who consumed a noncaffeinated sports drink, likely because caffeine speeds glucose absorption in the intestine. Other research shows that cyclists performed up to 23 percent more work during a time trial test after drinking a caffeinated beverage than they did after drinking a buzz-free beverage.

The best time to caffeinate is about 30 to 60 minutes before go time. Since you can overdo caffeine and end up jittery, keep the dose moderate. Research shows just 3 to 6 milligrams per kilogram of body weight is plenty. That's about 350 milligrams—the amount you'd get in a nice mug of coffee—for a 150-pound rider.

butter sandwich bits, fig bars, bananas, and the like before moving to energy bars, since consuming too many sugary sports foods (like bars and especially gels, blocks, and beans) can lead to gastrointestinal distress, or "gut rot" (see "Avoid Gut Rot," page 135) during long endurance events.

You can get some of your carbohydrate calories through sports drinks, though how many is a point of controversy. There are sports scientists who believe you can (and should) get the lion's share of your calories through liquid nutrition, such as specially formulated high-calorie drinks, so your mouth (which is low on saliva during exercise) and stomach (which is low on blood) don't have to work on digesting food. There's an opposing school of thought, though, that says you should limit the calories you get from fluids to less than 100 per hour. Scientists in this camp contend that you should instead put food in your pocket and hydration in your bottle. They believe the stomach can have trouble sorting out sugars (and carbs) from water, leaving you low on both.

Who's right? You might have to be the judge of that. Personally, I have used both approaches with success. The one problem with going the liquid calorie route is that you can end up in a bind if it's very hot and all you have are 400-calorie bottles. I learned that the hard way during a hot race in Africa, when I unwittingly sucked down about 800 calories of liquid nutrition in an hour or so because it was 97°F. I've never suffered so horribly for 50 miles. After that day, I reserved the high-calorie bottles for cooler events.

FLUIDS FOR THE RIDE

For years, cyclists were told they should drink enough during exercise so that they weigh the same when they rack their bike as they did when they saddled up and clicked in. But that's neither realistic nor necessary nor productive. Your body can't absorb the fluids as fast as you lose them. What's more, not every ounce of the weight you lose when you ride is lost through sweat. Some of the weight you lose comes from burned carbohydrate and fat stores, as well as the water that is stored with them. Those fluid losses don't contribute to dehydration or lower your blood volume. "You can lose one to two percent of your body weight and it won't hurt your performance," says Jeukendrup.

Ultimately, your goal should be to prevent performance-hindering dehydration. That means replacing about 75 percent of what you lose. "To do that, you need to know your sweat rate, which most cyclists underestimate," says sports nutrition expert Monique

Tapered and Loaded

A classic example of nutrient timing is the tried-and-true carbo-load, where you take a couple of days to fully load your glycogen stores before you unload them on the racecourse.

To do carbo-loading correctly, you need to dial back your training volume (so you aren't emptying out your glycogen stores) and skew your food intake so you're taking in proportionately more carbohydrates. You'll want to eat about 3 to 5 grams of carbohyrdates per pound of body weight during this time. That's 450 to 750 grams a day (where you aim on this scale depends on the duration of your event) for a 150-pound rider. A study published in the *International Journal of Sports Medicine* found that runners who consumed more than 7 grams of carbohydrates per kilogram of body weight (that's about 475 grams for a 150-pound rider) the day before their races posted significantly faster race times and maintained their running speeds better than those who ate fewer carbs.

Be aware that for every ounce of carbohydrate you store in your body, you store almost 3 ounces of water. That means that you'll likely gain about 1 to 3 pounds and feel a little like a bloated tick (never a fun feeling) going into race day. Don't let it get to your head. That's all just potential energy that you'll blow through by the time you get to the finish line, and you'll get there a whole lot faster for having stored it up.

Ryan, RD. Ryan, the author of *Sports Nutrition for Endurance Athletes*, recently coached a heavy-sweating triathlete who routinely lost 40 ounces of fluid—nearly two bottles' worth—an hour. To determine your sweat rate, weigh yourself before and after a short ride, suggests Ryan. "An hour ride is a good indicator of what you're losing through sweat alone."

In general, the recommendation to drain about a bottle an hour will keep you adequately hydrated. Unless the conditions are very hot and you're dripping sweat (in which case you do need additional fluids), drinking more won't speed you up and could actually slow you down. In a study from the Sports Science Institute of South Africa, researchers found that runners who drank at a high rate (about 10 ounces every 15 to 20 minutes) fared far worse (some couldn't even finish the test because of stomach upset) than those who drank at a moderate rate of 4 ounces every 14 to 20 minutes (a bottle an hour) or those who simply drank by thirst (about 13 ounces an hour).

Speaking of thirst, tune in to it. Contrary to what we used to be told (*drink, drink, drink!*), your thirst is a good guide, and your goal is simply to keep it at bay. By taking a few sips every 10 to 15 minutes as your mouth gets dry and you feel thirst, you'll stay hydrated and avoid the stomach upset that comes with guzzling a bottle at a time.

What to drink? Ultimately, as mentioned earlier, that's a personal preference that generally takes some trial and error to sort through. The one must-have for any drink, however, is electrolytes. Remember the "electrolyte bonk"? Electrolytes are critical for maintaining proper hydration. Choose a drink with sodium (about 400 to 600 milligrams per serving) as well as calcium and magnesium.

POSTRIDE REPLENISHMENT

Finishing a long hard ride or race without stocking your fuel stores is a bit like building a sand sculpture on the water's edge. All your hard work and effort can be washed away before you get to enjoy it. Remember, even if you've been faithfully fueling during your ride, you will finish in a semidepleted state. Your hardworking muscles also will be in need of repair.

Unless you refuel appropriately, your body will go into a catabolic state (meaning you'll be cannibalizing your lean muscle tissue—not good for getting faster). Your postride goal should be to switch from a catabolic to anabolic (*build, build, build!*) state as quickly as possible. That means you need protein within 20 minutes and carbohydrates very soon thereafter (if not simultaneously). For the best results, aim for about 20 to 30 grams of protein and 0.6 grams of carbohydrate per pound of body weight (around 90 grams for a 150-pound rider). One easy and tasty way to get the recovery fuel you need: 16 ounces of chocolate milk and a banana.

Restocking your glycogen stores and giving your muscles the amino acids they need to repair right away will help you get faster in the long run on two fronts. For one, you're ensuring a speedy recovery, so you can train hard again sooner and keep your results coming. Just as important, you're far less likely to overeat later in the day (and eventually pack on pounds).

Countdown to Fast

Dropping pounds to pick up speed.

There are very few cyclists I know who have no interest in losing at least a little (if not a lot of) weight. Whether we're coming out of the holiday season or a particularly busy time at work, nearly all of us at some time or another will pull on our spandex and think, "I could lose a few."

On paper, weight loss is a simple equation. You take in 500 fewer (or burn off 500 more) calories than you're currently taking in per day and you will lose a pound—3,500 calories in each—in a week's time. Were it only so simple, none of us would have an ounce to lose.

Scientists now know that weight loss is more than just a numbers game. Low-calorie foods can actually lead to weight gain, while high-calorie foods may help you take weight off. It's the composition that counts in this equation, because your body burns different fuel sources at different rates (and yes, those extra-large, sugar-soaked coffee beverages are a pretty bad idea).

Let's say you eat a 2,000-calorie diet composed mostly of your kid's cold cereals, plates of spaghetti, and frozen, processed chicken patties washed down with diet soda. You might not lose an ounce. In fact, you might put on a few. Now let's say you eat the same number of calories from whole oats and eggs, beans and rice, and salmon and sautéed vegetables. You may just lose more pounds than the classic equation would indicate.

"I have many clients who don't really make any changes to how many calories they eat on a given day, but we change the composition of those calories and they lose weight," says Anne Guzman, a sports nutrition consultant for the Peaks Coaching Group and former pro bike racer. Why? Because a calorie is not always a calorie. And that is the first rule of weight loss.

BURN AFTER EATING

A calorie is technically the unit of heat required to raise the temperature of 1 gram of water by 1 degree Celsius. (Scientists used to measure calories in food by setting them on fire . . . seriously.) Inside every cell you have mitochondria (power plants) that burn the food you eat to make energy for you to live. Just as coal burns differently from gas, which burns differently from a pile of tinder, so do proteins, fats, and carbohydrates burn differently within your body. Likewise, the kinds of proteins, fats, and carbohydrates you eat determine how much energy you store and burn . . . and how much weight you lose in the process.

In a nutshell, there are calories that are "active," which means your body uses lots of energy to digest them, and there are calories that are "lazy," which means they go straight to your bloodstream (and then to storage—i.e., fat) without much work.

Case in point, for every 100 calories of carbohydrates you eat, your body burns about 5 to 15 calories processing and digesting them. (More complex carbohydrates, such as brown rice and vegetables, burn the most; very fibrous foods burn up to 20 calories per 100.) Fats require very little energy, about 5 calories for every 100 you consume. Protein has the highest "thermic effect of food," as it's called. It scorches 20 to 30 out of every 100 calories for digestion.

For weight loss purposes, protein should be a priority at every meal (see how much you need on page 121). But don't shove all the rice off your plate as you make room for the chicken. Contrary to what some cyclists believe, piling on protein won't melt off pounds. "Typically the cyclists I see who are having trouble losing weight are eating too much protein and fat and too few carbs," says Guzman. As you saw in Chapter 8, where you calculated how many grams of each macronutrient you needed, balance is key because protein doesn't provide much energy for riding; you can't burn fat without carbs, and eating too little of any one thing leaves you depleted, while consuming too much of any one thing pads your fat stores.

Equally important is the form of your calorie intake. Look at what you're about to eat. Do you immediately recognize it as its original form in nature—a carrot, a grain, a slice of meat? Good. That is food at its finest, most active form. The more processing a food goes through—the less recognizable it is—the less your body has to work to digest it, the less satisfying it is, and the less useful it is for weight loss. The closer foods are to their natural state, the more fiber and water they have, which means they get digested slowly, leave you feeling satisfied with less, and provide longer-lasting energy.

A study published in *Food and Nutrition Research* compared the thermic effect of food of two cheese sandwich lunches that were identical in calories, protein, fat, and carbohydrates, but were composed of either processed foods (white bread, processed cheese) or whole foods (multigrain bread, cheddar cheese). The average post-meal energy expenditure of the whole food meal was *twice as high* (20 percent of the meal's calories) as that of the processed meal (just over 10 percent of the meal's calories).

I cowrote a book titled *The Active Calorie Diet* based on this science with sports nutritionist Leslie Bonci, MPH, RD, director of sports nutrition at the Center for Sports Medicine at the University of Pittsburgh Medical Center. Bonci's clients who adopted the book's plan were very successful for one simple reason. "Just by changing the composition of your plate, you can get very close to the recommended amounts of all the macronutrients you need and start losing weight without taking a single additional step," says Bonci. "Structuring your meals this way will allow you to ride well and fill up, but not out."

GET LEAN, GET FAST! PLATE

One-quarter to one-third of the plate should be active calories from protein such as lean meat, skinless poultry, fish, soy foods, eggs, or low-fat dairy.

One-half of the plate should be active calories from fruits/vegetables.

One-quarter of the plate should be active calories from whole grain starches such as brown rice, whole wheat pasta, potatoes, and tortillas.

Minimize lazy calories by saving them for occasional indulgences and/or snacks.

Active Calories

Fruits

Vegetables

Whole grains

Beans and legumes

Lean meat, fish, poultry

Fiber-rich cereal

Whole grain bread

Dairy foods

Soups

Lazy Calories

Pastries, cookies, pies, and cakes

Processed meats

Chips, pretzels, and snack foods

Fast food such as burgers, chicken patties, and french fries

BALANCING YOUR BUDGET

Like your checking and savings accounts, the best way to manage calories (and your weight) is to balance them. If you have just a little weight to lose, following the food-intake advice from Chapter 8, the timing advice from Chapter 9, and the plate-partitioning advice above will get you there. If you have more than, say, 10 pounds to lose and/or you have a history of struggling with your weight, keeping track of your calories in and calories out will help you run a little into the red and finally shed the unwanted baggage.

The trick is learning how, says Bonci. "There's an awful lot of human error when it comes to calorie management. Unless every morsel you eat has a food label—and you know exactly how much you're eating—it's difficult to know how much you're taking in. It can be even harder to know how much you're burning." Researchers have found that exercisers tend to overestimate how many calories their sweat sessions burn—sometimes by nearly 1,000, or about a half a day's worth.

The total number you came up with in Chapter 8 should put you very close to your target daily calorie intake, including the food calories you burn on your bike. For a frame of reference, pedaling your bike burns about 9 to 10 calories per minute. Ballpark about 500 calories an hour for a 150-pound rider. If you're heavier, you burn more; if you're lighter, you burn less.

Now for the other side of the equation—figuring out how many calories you're taking in. It's easy when every food you eat has a label. But, especially if you're eating fresh, nonpackaged foods as advised, that's just often not the case. Here your best bet is to turn to an online calorie calculator or download one of the many free food- and exercise-tracking apps. These services make calorie counting pretty painless by putting enormous food databases at your fingertips. All you do is punch in the food and it pops up, complete with nutrient breakdown. Plug in the amount and you're done. Most of these services also offer a fitness log component so you can track what you're burning as well. (Of course, if you use a power meter, you can get these numbers on every ride.)

A Sample Get Fast! Day

I asked a few sports nutritionists to give me a snapshot of an ideal day of eating to Get Fast! The results were all pretty similar. If you're looking to lose weight, it's about 2,200 calories for active cyclists. And it breaks down like this sample day from Anne Guzman, a sports nutrition consultant for the Peaks Coaching Group.

Morning preride snack: banana drizzled with honey

Breakfast: oatmeal with nut butter and fruit

Midmorning snack: hummus and baby carrots

Lunch: grilled chicken sandwich with fresh greens and mustard on whole grain bread

Afternoon snack: an apple, some orange slices, and a handful of almonds

Dinner: grilled turkey burger with oven-baked sweet potato fries and sautéed spinach

On the bike: sports drink, fig bars or an energy bar

Fast Diet Tips

Researchers estimate that you make more than 200 food decisions each day. Each one has the power to tip the scales in your favor. Here are 10 fast diet tips that will keep the pounds coming off.

1. Skip the Diet Soda

Research has been mounting for the past 15 years that artificial sweeteners don't work for weight loss. In fact, they seem to backfire. In one nearly decade-long study, researchers found that those who drank two or more diet drinks a day had waistline increases 500 percent greater than non-diet-soda drinkers. Aspartame seems to raise blood sugar levels and leave you craving more starch and sugar. Stick to seltzer.

2. Get Pickled and Spiced

Fermented foods such as yogurt, sauerkraut, and pickles promote healthy digestion and nutrient absorption. Spices such as ginger and hot peppers spike your metabolism. Both help temper cravings for sweets.

3. Think Thirst First

It's very easy to mistake a little dehydration for hunger. Grab a thirst-quenching drink before you raid the fridge.

4. Keep the Calories Coming

It can be tempting to pull out the stops and starve yourself for a few days to hit fighting weight, but resist the urge. All you'll lose is water weight (remember how glycogen stores water with it; as you rip through your carb stores, the water goes, too). Worse, if you keep that self-induced famine up too long, your body will reset its metabolism so it burns fewer calories to perform the basic daily functions of staying alive. That means as soon as you start to eat normally again, the pounds you lost—and likely a few extra—will pile back on.

5. Weigh In

All those decisions are easier to make when you see progress . . . or lack thereof. The National Weight Control Registry shows that one of the top habits of successful "losers" is they monitor their weight regularly. Step on the scale every Monday morning.

6. Turn Down the Tap

No one (especially not me) is going to tell you to give up beer or your favorite boozy beverage. Just keep alcohol consumption to a minimum. When you drink alcohol, your body burns that first, so you burn less fat and you burn it more slowly than usual. Tipping back two martinis is enough to slow your fat-burning ability by about 73 percent. And those buffalo wings look better and better after each beer.

7. Befriend Your Farmer's Market

When possible, choose organic produce and free-range meats (especially grass-fed beef). For one, the nutritional profiles are healthier. Grass-fed beef is lower in fat—just 2.5 grams per 4 ounces, compared to nearly 11 grams in 4 ounces of grain-fed cattle—and has considerably more metabolism-revving omega-3 fatty acids and less saturated fat than corn-fed cows. Organic foods are also free of toxins that may interfere with your weight loss. Researchers at Laval University in Quebec City found that pesticides like those used on nonorganic produce can leach into your system and interfere with the energy-

burning process, leading to a metabolic slowdown as you lose weight.

8. Tea Up

I love coffee as much as the next cyclist, but swapping your third or fourth (or fifth) cup of joe for a big mug of green tea may help your metabolism keep humming along in high gear. According to one Japanese study, a cup of brewed tea can boost your fat metabolism by 12 percent.

9. Put It on Ice

Drinking about 6 cups of water can fire up your resting metabolism by about 50 calories per day, according to research. Not a monumental amount, but enough to take off 5 pounds at the end of a year. Add ice for an even bigger metabolic bump. Your body has to work to warm the water, which burns another additional 10 calories. It all adds up.

10. Spin Fasted

Get on your trainer or rollers for 20 minutes before you eat breakfast. You'll crank up your fat-burning metabolism and start the day off right.

Some reputable (and free) sites to check out include SparkPeople, My-Calorie-Counter, FitDay, and MyNetDiary. Study after study shows that logging your food is the most effective way to lose weight. Why? I believe it's because it makes you mindful of what you're eating and prevents you from housing a bag of chips, because nobody wants to type that into their food log.

For the best results, I recommend using logging as an educational process. Give yourself a month. Log your food. Log your exercise. Build in a small daily indulgence (this shouldn't be punishment, after all). Make notes about the foods that give you the most energy. Write down improvements you notice in your riding. Pay close attention to what appropriate portions look like. See how you feel and how much weight you lose by the end of 4 weeks.

When you're losing weight as you'd like and you're confident that you've gotten the feel for how to balance your calorie budget, start weaning yourself off the tracking system and just continue eating and riding the way you've been. If the pounds start creeping back up, you can always return to logging to get back on track.

11

Supplemental Speed

Get Fast! pills, potions, and powders— what really works.

Fast Fact: Athletes around the globe (including those of the weekend warrior variety) spent a record $31.2 billion on sports supplements in 2008. By the time this book reaches your hands, that number is projected to soar to $91.8 billion, according to BCC Research, a Massachusetts-based market analysis and research firm.

In the early days before GNC, Competitive Cyclist, and Joe Weider, our active ancestors wolfed down lion hearts, elk livers, and coca leaves to gain strength, speed, and competitive advantage. Those ergogenic aids were primitive, sure. But like all good folk medicine, they weren't without scientific merit. Today, sales of creatine powder (a protein-like substance that lion hearts would be loaded with) top $14 million in the United States alone. Ephedra (not unlike coca leaves) continues to rack up Internet sales despite having being causally linked to some serious health complications.

Cyclists are particularly eager to eat up anything that promises to make them fast, lean, and strong. But what's the real deal, and what's more bull than Rocky Mountain oysters? Honestly, it's hard to know sometimes. Many a sports supplement has passed through the *Bicycling* magazine offices over the years. For a while, we had a column called Lab Rat where we reviewed all the latest (if not greatest) potions and pills. It fizzled out, not for lack of product, but for lack of promise. There just wasn't enough to say about the majority of them. Nearly everything seemed to have some benefits for some people. Nothing worked for everyone. And it was all pretty difficult to quantify. Even the most gold standard double-blind research studies were rarely conclusive.

That said, there are some supplements out there that stand up pretty well under scientific scrutiny, as well as those that many cyclists and cycling coaches swear by. Here's a look at a few that might help make you faster. But remember, before you spend a dime, take care of the big stuff first. Train hard. Eat a healthy diet. Sleep 8 hours a night. And upgrade old clunky components. That stuff is the meat and potatoes of performance. Supplements are pure gravy. Use as directed.

WHEY PROTEIN

Hard, long rides break down muscle tissue and can lead to prolonged soreness and fatigue. The amino acids in protein build them back up. The faster you feed them the protein they need, the more quickly and completely they'll repair (and the less sore you'll be). For the quickest amino acid delivery service, slug down some whey protein. Whey, the naturally occurring protein in milk, is considered one of the best proteins for muscle repair because the body can absorb and use it very quickly—some experts say within 15 minutes—so recovery time is shortened. Some researchers believe that whey protein also reduces oxidative stress from free radicals produced during exercise, which also may reduce subsequent muscle fatigue. Recently, a study of 20 competitive male cyclists reported that supplementing with whey protein increased their lymphocyte (white blood cells critical for immunity) levels, which could prevent you from getting sick during hard training and racing blocks.

Stacy Sims, PhD, a Stanford-based exercise physiologist and nutrition scientist with Osmo Nutrition, recommends whey protein before and after hard training. "You want a protein load before and after training to boost muscle adaptations. Your pre-workout snack could be a scoop of whey isolate protein powder, espresso, water (iced protein latte!). The caffeine and protein will boost your training sessions, allowing you to get more power adaptations from your sessions. Post-workout, you have a thirty-minute window for protein, up to two hours for carbohydrate. An ideal recovery drink is six to eight ounces of low-fat chocolate milk," she says. As a bonus, the bit of sugar will stimulate the release of insulin, which will help shuttle glucose into your hungry cells for complete recovery.

In a recent study, researchers from the University of Texas at Austin had 32 volunteers cycle 60 minutes a day, 5 days a week for $4\frac{1}{2}$ weeks. Those who drank chocolate milk post-pedaling enjoyed greater VO_2 max gains and better body composition changes than those who drank a plain carb beverage. Chocolate milk—maybe the tastiest supplement ever.

BETA-ALANINE

This might be one of the best sports supplements you've never heard of. Beta-alanine is an amino acid that is naturally produced by the body and is readily used by your fast-twitch muscles for sprinting fuel. The supplement cracked the cycling scene a few years ago when a study of 25 cyclists reported that those taking the supplement improved their scores in a cycling performance test by 13 percent after just 4 weeks. A follow-up study was equally promising. This time, riders who took about 6 grams a day for 4 weeks improved their time to exhaustion in a full-throttle cycling test by more than 12 percent. Those taking just a dummy pill improved just 1.6 percent on the test.

Sims has recommended it for years. "It improves muscle fiber firing rate and recovery," she says. Research has shown improvements with dosages of between 3.2 and 6.4 grams a day. You can find beta-alanine as a stand-alone supplement or bundled with other ingredients in sports supplements such as OptygenHP (see page 156).

OMEGA-3

While not necessarily a "sports supplement," omega-3 fatty acids deliver many important benefits that can help you stay healthy and get faster on your bike. Most important, they reduce inflammation. Omega-3s also keep your heart healthy by controlling blood pressure and triglycerides. Some studies suggest they might also help with weight loss. The government recommends that adults eat at least two servings of fatty fish a week to meet omega-3 needs. But frankly, for active folks like cyclists, that doesn't really cut it. Far too few people eat that much fish anyway.

"Omega-3s are the one time I tell people to just go ahead and take a pill, because so few of us get enough from food," says sports nutritionist Leslie Bonci, MPH, RD, director of sports nutrition at the Center for Sports Medicine at the University of Pittsburgh Medical Center. "Aim for one thousand to two thousand milligrams a day, especially when you're training, because you're generating more inflammation, which is detrimental to your overall health as well as recovery."

TEA EXTRACTS

Green tea has been hailed as somewhat of a panacea over the years, with claims that it prevents and/or cures everything from heart disease to cancer to obesity. Well, some scientists also believe it may just make you faster by boosting your endurance. Animal studies have found that the equivalent of four cups of green tea a day improved endurance in a swimming test by up to 25 percent. That level of performance boost hasn't been replicated in humans. But we do know that the catechins in green tea enhance fat metabolism, so they also may help you ride stronger longer before hitting the wall.

Black tea extracts also may improve your riding, according to sports scientists at Rutgers University, who found that a 9-day supplement of black tea extract decreased muscle soreness and improved recovery following high intensity cycling intervals. In an interview with *Bicycling* magazine, lead study author Shawn Arent, PhD, explained, "The black tea extract reduces oxidative stress of the exercises and speeds recovery between intervals." You can make some yourself by steeping four bags of decaffeinated tea in 32 ounces of cold water overnight, says Barbara Lewin, RD, of Sports-Nutritionist.com. Sip it before, during, and after rides.

ARGININE

Here's a promising one for the masters in the room. Researchers reporting in the *Journal of the International Society of Sports Nutrition* gave a group of cyclists between ages 50 and 73 either arginine supplements or dummy pills for 1 week and then tested their anaerobic thresholds (the level of work they need to do before lactic acid begins to accumulate). Those taking the arginine supplements saw an impressive 16.7 percent increase in their thresholds.

Arginine works by supporting the nitric oxide (NO) system, which stimulates the blood vessels around the heart and other organs to dilate and helps increase exercise capacity. As we age, our production of NO declines and takes our exercise performance with it. Nitric oxide is created from arginine, so supplementing seems to stave off this decline. Amino Vital is a popular supplemental source of arginine. As a bonus, it also contains other branched-chain amino acids (BCAAs), such as L-glutamine, which is believed to help boost immunity and protect against symptoms of overtraining. It makes for a good second bottle on a long ride, or a primary hydration source if you also pack a gel or bar.

OPTYGENHP

Here's one that's a favorite among *Bicycling* magazine staffers (myself included). The manufacturer, First Endurance, also supplies OptygenHP to a number of pro teams including HTC-Highroad, RadioShack Nissan Trek, and Specialized-lululemon.

OptygenHP is a blend supplement, so it contains a number of active ingredients, including the mineral chromium, the herbal extract *Cordyceps sinensis*, beta-alanine (see page 154), and rhodiola, an herb long used by Tibetan Sherpas to improve their endurance and ability to use oxygen. Rhodiola is an adaptogen, which means it helps your body adapt to stresses. The scientific jury is still out on rhodiola, as there are about an equal number of studies showing its benefits as there are showing just the opposite.

Those who use OptygenHP claim that it makes hard training feel easier and allows them to train and race hard repeatedly with less recovery time. This is a "load-and-sustain" supplement: You take this stuff every day (four a day with meals), and long term. First Endurance claims little to no benefits if you start taking it immediately before exercise.

SPORTLEGS

Here's another one you'll find in the medicine cabinets of many fellow *Bicycling* magazine staffers (yes, it's in mine, too). The special ingredient here is the lactate forms of calcium and magnesium. Yep, lactate, like the stuff that your body produces when you're working really hard. Your body uses lactate as a buffer to slow down the acidosis that occurs during high-intensity exercise (which is what actually causes the burn). SportLegs preloads your legs with lactate.

The supplement itself has not been studied on athletes, but the individual ingredients have been studied with success. SportLegs also has stood up to one of the biggest tests: time. The supplement entered the cycling market in the fall of 2002 and has been selling strongly ever since. Nearly everyone who tries it says the same thing: SportLegs just makes you feel like you're having a good day on the bike. SportLegs loyalists feel like they can push past the point where they'd normally feel like they were shutting down.

What's especially nice about this supplement is that you don't need to take it all the time for it to work. Just pop a few capsules (one per every 50 pounds of body weight) an hour before your ride and you're good to go. On long rides, multiday rides, and races, riders often carry a small bag with some pills so they can reload every 2 to 3 hours.

ACID CHECK

Being too acidic is a bad thing for sports performance. Unfortunately, we all become a little more acidic over time because of age-related kidney changes. Our blood acid/alkaline balance tips into the acid direction and we excrete nitrogen, an essential component of muscle protein, faster than we take it in. That's bad because we can't form new muscle and our recovery grinds to a halt. You can turn the tide on nitrogen loss and preserve your muscles (and speed your recovery) by increasing the alkalinity of your blood. A healthy diet (rich in fruits and veggies) goes a long way in providing that "neutral support," so to speak. You also can buy supplements such as Acid Check to help you along.

Made with calcium and magnesium along with potassium, this supplement also provides the same threshold-bumping benefit that SportLegs does. Acid Check's mineral cocktail, which its manufacturer has patented as Alka-Myte, has been studied on animals and humans and was found to increase time to exhaustion, lower the level of acid in the blood, and improve muscle recovery rates. Unlike the manufacturers of SportLegs, the makers of Acid Check recommend daily use for the best results.

CAFFEINE

You don't need a pill or powder to reap the rewards of this perennial power booster. As cyclists, we base entire rides around our favorite caffeine vendors. As mentioned in Chapter 10, you don't need much to enjoy a performance jolt. Just 3 to 6 milligrams per kilogram of body weight about an hour before go time does the trick. In plain English, that's a 10-ounce mug of drip for a typical 150-pound rider.

If you're not a coffee drinker, there are plenty of other sources, such as those 5-Hour Energy shots (which also contain B vitamins), that deliver about 200 milligrams of caffeine and are pretty convenient to stash in a jersey pocket for those extended days on the bike.

Interestingly, there's mounting scientific evidence that caffeine may also help accelerate glycogen replacement when you take it immediately after a workout. I personally like to make a recovery mocha out of 1 or 2 percent milk, chocolate milk powder, and a shot or two of espresso.

The Track Stack

When I was preparing to go race the Breck Epic (the 6-day mountain bike stage race in Breckenridge, Colorado), I pinged my go-to nutrition source, Stanford-based exercise physiologist and nutrition scientist Stacy Sims, for some last-minute nutrition tips. The one that stuck: the Track Stack, a modified supplement concoction she recommends taking 20 minutes before the gun goes off to prime the pump.

It's a modification of the old bodybuilding and track racing stack, says Sims. The original stack was aspirin, caffeine, ephedrine, and sometimes nitric oxide. She modified the blend to give the same effects but to *not* damage any organs, since ephedrine damages the heart and nitric oxide damages natural vessel compliance and feedback. As mentioned earlier, beta-alanine aids muscle firing. It also works as a vasodilator, like nitric oxide.

THE TRACK STACK*

150 mg of caffeine (stimulant)

2 x 81 mg of baby aspirin (dilates blood vessels)

2,000 mg of beta-alanine (improves muscle fiber firing rate)

* This dose is for riders in the 155- to 175-pound range. Smaller riders should cut the dose to 100 mg of caffeine, 1 x 81 mg of baby aspirin, and 1,500 mg of beta-alanine.

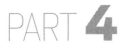
PART **4**

THINK FAST
Go as fast as you put your mind to going.

I didn't win Kona on my physical prowess. I won it with my mind being able to override my body. Mental strength is key. No amount of physical strength will help you win if you don't have what it takes to be mentally driven and focused. You need to be able to relax and stay in the moment and endure boredom and have a load of positive images to carry with you. All those things are what help you win.

—Chrissie Wellington

I've always been firmly convinced that when all else is equal—and let's face it, so often we are on the line with many folks who are pretty equal to us in strength and speed—what wins races isn't your legs. It's your head.

How you think. What you think. Whether you tune in or tune out. How you talk to yourself. The images in your head. How you react to competition. How you manage stress. How you prepare mentally and how well you care for and train your brain have as much a bearing on how fast you can go as any intervals, gym work, or periodic training plan.

World champions like Chrissie Wellington stay on top of their game by using their heads. And studies are showing that the power of brain training isn't just their imagination.

SEND YOURSELF INTO OVERDRIVE

Among the most compelling bits of new research to come out on the power of the mind is a study out of England that found that scientists could trick cyclists into beating their own personal bests simply by telling them they were going slower than they really were.

In the study, British researchers had a group of cyclists repeatedly perform a $2\frac{1}{2}$-mile time trial on a stationary trainer as fast as they could muster over a period of days to clock their absolute best time. Then they asked half the group to perform the time trial again, this time against a computer-generated avatar that they thought was pacing their personal best record on the course, while it was in fact set to go at a pace that was 1 percent faster (producing about 2 percent more power) than the rider's fastest time. The other half of the group was told they would, in fact, be racing a faster avatar. You can guess what happened. The riders who thought they were matching their best set PRs, while those who thought they were outclassed couldn't keep up.

You can use that knowledge to tap into hidden potential. Find a slightly stronger friend (not one that can dust you, as that can be counterproductive) and make it your goal to match them. Most important, *believe you can*. The researchers speculate that ultimately, optimum performance is ruled by your belief system and how your brain paces you based on that. "Confidence is so critical when the pain and the inner voices build during a competition performance. It is self-belief that pushes you on," says study researcher Kevin Thompson, a fellow at the British Association of Sport and Exercise Sciences.

Still not convinced? As you'll see later in this section, other research found that men and women who just *imagined* exercising their biceps 5 days a week for 12 weeks boosted their strength by more than 13 percent, though they never actually moved a muscle, while those who did no imaginary exercise reaped no strength gains. How is that possible? It's your mind-muscle connection again. "When you visualize an action, your brain maps it out in your body, so your muscles are primed to perform," says Sean McCann, PhD, sports psychologist with the US Olympic Training Center in Colorado Springs.

Think about it. You spend season after season logging enough base miles to have lungs like hot air balloons and capillary beds that resemble black widow colonies. But what have you done for your head? When all things are equal, the rider who is the most mentally fit finishes first; yet few of us ever bother training our brain, says Paige Dunn, former sports psychology consultant for Clif Bar and Company and founder of Xcel Sport Psychology Group in Oakland, California. "Mental strength is what sets you apart as an athlete. You can be the most physically fit athlete, but if you are not mentally prepared, you will not perform your best."

The takeaway here is that you are faster than you think. You can go faster and farther than you know. Even when you think you've given it all you've got, there's a little bit more inside. It's time to learn how to let it out. This section will show you how.

12

Mind over Muscles

Train your brain and your legs will follow.

Fast Fact: Exercisers working out to music can increase their endurance by up to 15 percent and their speed and performance by as much as 20 percent compared to those who move in silence. "Music blocks fatigue; produces feelings of vigor, happiness, and excitement; and can help you keep pace as you synchronize your movements to the music," says Costas Karageorghis, PhD, of the Brunel University School of Sport and Education in West London.

If how fast and how far you could ride was determined by your physical prowess alone, putting your favorite playlist in your ear would make a nice soundtrack, but it wouldn't speed you up. In reality, however, the amount of power we can put into our pedals is determined every bit as much by the "muscle" between our ears as it is by the ones pushing our gears.

Turning up a little Rage Against the Machine is only one way to unleash the power of your mind to override your muscles. Top athletes use a whole arsenal of mental tools and tricks such as visualization, self-talk, and breath control to push through pain, break performance barriers, and tap into unharnessed speed. Here's what you need to know.

TALK NICE

Something about pushing through searing quad pain and gasping for the next breath can make you start talking to yourself. And the conversation is often unpleasant, sometimes downright hostile. Studies show both negative and positive self-talk influence performance. You can guess which one works best. A recent meta-analysis of 32 sports psychology studies confirmed that motivational self-talk, like "I am strong; I can do this," can significantly improve endurance performance. Also helpful is instructional positive self-talk, like "spin perfect circles," which keeps you mindful of maintaining good technique.

"When you say, 'Oh, no. Here comes the hill. This is going to hurt,' it will. Worse than it would without the negative self-talk," says Paige Dunn, former sports psychology consultant for Clif Bar and Company and founder of Xcel Sport Psychology Group in Oakland, California. "Catastrophizing greatly increases your sense of pain," adds Sean McCann, PhD, sports psychologist with the US Olympic Training Center in Colorado Springs. "Be very careful about how you talk to yourself. If you say, 'Oh my God, this is the terrible. I'm dying,' you'll suffer worse."

In fact, some scientists believe that as soon as the negative thoughts creep in, you're as good as done. "You have to make the decision. You have to believe it. Once you start doubting, you change your brain chemistry and you're done," explained South African researcher Timothy Noakes, MD, during a conversation on his life-long theories on fatigue. Noakes is the longtime champion of the "central governor" theory of fatigue, which in short says that your brain is the one calling the shots and shutting you down, even when you have plenty of fuel in the tank and untapped muscle fibers in your legs.

The central governor starts its job the moment you clip in, metering out your efforts based on your training, previous experience, the duration ahead, your metabolic state, and information it's gathering from your heart, muscles, and parts of the brain. As mentioned earlier, studies have shown that even when riders bonk or fail to finish a ride (DNF) from seemingly insurmountable fatigue, they still have glycogen stores and fresh muscle fibers at their disposal. The governor, for other reasons, simply decided it was best to not go on. It's a protective mechanism. But also—in some instances—perhaps an overprotective mechanism.

As soon as you start talking negatively, you're giving the governor the green light to flick the off switch because it's sensing that things aren't going so well. Instead, give yourself a mental (and physical) boost up those inclines with words that lift you up.

Think, "Relax. Spin fast and easy," or "Smooth perfect circles will take me to the top." Or do what I do and downplay the difficulty of the situation. When the pavement kicks up, for instance, I say, "The hill is flat," over and over. Sure, it's a lie, but according to Peter Terry, coauthor of *Inside Sport Psychology*, lying to yourself works just fine. "Self-talk plays an influential role in endurance performance. Even if we know that the hill isn't really flat, telling ourselves that it is can reduce the negative effects of anxiety, keep our minds firmly on the task at hand, and provide a much-needed boost to self-belief. Most people are pretty suggestible, even to the point of choosing fantasy over reality." Works for me.

Terry and his coauthor, Costas Karageorghis, offer other self-talk cues to use to control your mood when your mental state threatens to trip you up. Jacked up with aggression? Try telling yourself, "Use it, don't lose it." Feeling sluggish? Say, "Eyes wide open." The possibilities are endless. Nervous? Go with "I am prepared." Use these simple phrases and mantras to quiet your mind and focus all your energy on the task at hand—riding strong and fast.

SEE YOURSELF SUCCEED

Everything you do from flipping the pages in this book to carving a corner through your favorite hometown crit comes down to your mind telling your muscles what to do. Turns out the more you mentally rehearse those movements (well, perhaps not necessary for turning pages), the more seamless they'll be in real life.

The power of mental imagery is so profound it can engage muscle fibers you're not even moving. Scientists from the Cleveland Clinic Foundation found that men and women who just *imagined* exercising their little finger and biceps 5 days a week for 12 weeks improved their strength by 53 percent and 13.4 percent, respectively, compared to zero gains among a similar group who did no imaginary exercise.

Likewise, French researchers recently found that volunteers who mentally rehearsed specific movements improved their performance even if they didn't physically practice. It's the product of your mind's mapping ability. When you visualize an action, your mind creates a blueprint for how to execute it. "That allows you to recruit the muscles you need and perform more effectively and efficiently when you actually do it. Elite-level athletes harness the power of visualization all the time," says McCann. Dunn agrees: "Come race day, you're almost on autopilot because you've practiced everything you need to do over and over and over in your mind."

Multitime mountain biking world champion Rebecca Rusch lives and breathes visualization when she tackles gut-busting, mind-bending ultraendurance challenges like the Leadville Trail 100, a 100-mile mountain bike race that soars into thin air territories over 12,000 feet in elevation in the Colorado Rockies. "I absolutely visualize sections of the course and especially the finish line in the weeks coming up to the big event," she says. "My second and third years at Leadville, I rode the last few blocks up Sixth Street and through the finish line multiple times before the race, imagining the red carpet, the crowd, and the time on the clock. Each of those times, I rode faster than the time I'd imagined and won the race."

She even visualizes in her driveway. "At home, I regularly ride into my cul-de-sac at the finish of a ride and put my hands in the air as I cross into the driveway. It's my own little mini finish line and also a positive affirmation to myself for doing my workout that day," she says.

Try it yourself. Whether you're preparing for a cyclocross race or just your next workout, take a few minutes to map it out in your mind. Start strong, clipping in without hesitation. Charge off the line. Sit and spin smooth, powerful circles. Stay calm and loose, flow with the pack, hold your line sure and steady through the corners, pedaling out of each one, keeping up your speed and momentum, standing and powering up short punchy rises, and feeling strong. Draw the most vivid picture imaginable and see it happen again and again.

Don't be afraid to visualize "bad" scenarios as well. Punctures happen. Mechanicals happen. So does panic if you let your head get the best of you. This is where you can call in tip one: Talk Nice (no sense kicking yourself when you're down). You can also visualize yourself going through the most common trouble scenarios. See yourself remaining calm, pulling out the tools you need, fixing the problem, and getting on with your race.

SUFFER GREATLY

One of my all-time favorite interviews was with John Stamstad, the godfather of solo ultraendurance mountain biking, who famously raced 23 hours of the 24 Hours of Canaan relay race in West Virginia with a compressed vertebra following a crash. We talked about pain, and specifically how he manages to suffer through so much so successfully.

"It took me a long time to stop treating pain like some horrible villain to be avoided," he told me. Instead, he started seeking it out and deciphering what it meant in various riding situations. "The worst thing to do is get emotional about your pain, because that heightens your sensations," said the man who once rode the final 80 miles of a 101-mile race with a broken collarbone. "Take it as a signal from your nervous system that you're working hard. And when you work hard, you do well." Back in the day, he would judge his pain based on his heart rate. If he was at 190 beats per minute (bpm)—damn close to max—and he was suffering, he was happy because it meant he was right where he needed to be. But if he was suffering at say, 165, he would take that as a cue to eat or hydrate. "If you listen to your pain unemotionally, it will help you," he said.

"People underestimate their pain threshold—and overestimate everyone else's," adds Dunn. "Everyone is suffering, not just you. Those who deal with their pain best acknowledge it for what it is and move past it." In other words, when your quads scream, turn your focus to the task at hand—pedaling your bike as fast as possible. "Stay in control of your thoughts; you can take more than you think when you keep your mind on your mission," says Dunn. "Tell yourself, 'This is how I feel when I go fast,'" adds McCann. "'This is how I feel when I win.' By framing your pain in a positive way, you manage the suffering without so much *suffering*."

If you can, take your turn at the front when the going gets really rough. "Control is one of the biggest keys to pain tolerance. If you feel it's out of your control, it hurts a lot more," says McCann. "When riding in a group, try to stay with the front riders. When you're in the back, it's easy to feel like the other guys are beating you down. When you're in the front, even if you're moving at the same pace, you automatically feel like you're the one punishing them."

Suffering is also a skill you can practice. "I practice my suffering ability in events all the time," says Rusch, who is aptly known as the Queen of Pain. "Situations that are especially trying, such as bad weather, broken equipment, getting lost, getting hurt and digging your way out of these holes, are all lessons that stay with me and then make other situations when the shit doesn't hit the fan seem easier. I've actually wished for bad weather in mountain bike races because I know that people without my background of being cold, lost, and hungry in the middle of the night wither at the thought of a bit of cold rain or snow. I know in these situations (like the first year I did Leadville) that I can excel by just putting my head down and pushing through."

Like Stamstad, Rusch has also practiced tuning in to that pain so she knows what she can take. "I try to embrace the pain and tell myself that I'm better at managing pain than my competitors," she says. "This comes with relaxing and accepting instead of fighting against it. I know that the sooner I get to the finish, the sooner the pain will stop. I remind myself that everything that's been worthwhile in my life has involved pain, suffering, and hard work. It makes the reward that much sweeter. Discovering that is powerful and addictive."

Indeed, some scientists believe that the suffering in and of itself is part of the reward of sport. The modern desk jockey existence is so devoid of punishing physical work that we seek outlets for pushing ourselves. In one scientific paper published in the journal *Leisure Studies*, sociologist Michael Atkinson, PhD, argues that many of us are on a quest for "exciting significance" in our lives through endurance sports (he was writing about triathlons specifically, but our sport certainly counts). He notes that we come together in a "mutually recognized pain community of like-minded actors," and that we relish the physical suffering as one of the primary rewards. When you look at it that way, it's not so bad . . . or at least it's worth it.

CHECK YOUR BRAIN

High-speed descents are called "scary fast" for a reason—they can leave even the best bike handlers shaking in their boots because your brain starts thinking of all the catastrophic things that could occur at those speeds.

Unfortunately, once you start thinking, or overthinking, the odds of said catastrophic things occurring increase as you tense up and start fighting the bike instead of flowing with it. This is especially true when you're on rough terrain, as when you're riding on gravel roads or mountain biking.

Of course you shouldn't be out there riding over your head. But don't let your head get in the way of riding as fast as you comfortably can, either. My all-time favorite mental trick for checking your head comes from nine-time US national mountain bike champion Leigh Donovan. When a race got hairy—or worse, she'd just crashed and lost her focus—she would count. Counting requires just enough concentration that it pushes out other thoughts that can otherwise rush in and occupy your brain. "I'll grab a number out of the air and start counting up or down—five, ten, fifteen, twenty—it quiets your mind and lets you get focused quickly," she says. Try it. It really works.

TAKE A DEEP BREATH

Control your breathing and you control your mind. If you're standing on the line—or worse, in the heat of battle—with a case of out of control stress, you're going to slow down, because rampant anxiety causes you to tense up and take shallow breaths, stealing energy. The single best way to quell stress and regain (or better yet, maintain) control is by breathing, says Dunn. "I have my athletes do 'circle breathing' before a competition or any time they feel stressed out. It helps them focus and center themselves. It's physiologically impossible to be freaking out while you perform it."

Inhale deeply and slowly through your nose, feeling your chest expand from top to bottom, finally allowing your abdomen to push fully outward. Pause. Then steadily exhale through your mouth, pushing out that last bit of breath so your belly fully hollows. Feel your muscles relax. Repeat 5 to 10 times.

Likewise, when you're on your bike, make deep breathing a habit. Concentrate on breathing deep into your body, pushing the abdominal part of your lungs down and out. Your abs should expand as much if not more than your chest. Check out Tour riders as they work their way up a long, steep climb. You'll see that their bellies expand and contract as they breathe. That not only makes the most of lung capacity, it serves the dual purpose of keeping you calm and in control.

Some riders like to synchronize their breathing to their pedal stroke, which respiratory researcher Paul Davenport, PhD, of the

University of Florida says may yield a small bump in performance. "Try falling into a cadence where you're exhaling at the top of your pedal strokes, alternating legs, pushing out your air to the rhythm of your effort. You're less likely to take incomplete breaths, and your effort will feel more even," he says. I like doing this on ridiculously steep mountain bike climbs because it helps me stay focused on the task at hand, ensures I breathe deeply, and occupies my mind, so the negative thoughts stay away.

CONTROL YOUR CONTROLLABLES

Top performance comes from confidence—confidence that you've prepared and have everything you need to ride or race well. Proper training is only a fraction of that equation. If you assume everyone else is out riding as much or more than you are, what sets you apart is all your other preparation.

Develop a system that allows you to gear up, train, race, and track and analyze your results in a systematic way that doesn't have you scurrying around looking for tools, tubes, spare cleats, pumps, and trying to remember the pressure you run in your tubulars when it's wet out.

When everything is where it's supposed to be and you know you have everything you need, the rest falls into place much more easily and you can focus every ounce of energy on your ride. It also gives you that much needed sense of control when it's so easy to feel out of control.

TUNE IN AND ZONE OUT

Costas Karageorghis describes music as a "legal drug for athletes." That's hard to argue with when you consider that it reduces your perceived effort, increases endurance, and distracts your mind from the fatigue you feel, allowing you to maintain hard efforts longer than you would in silence.

In short, music can help put you in and keep you in the zone—that seemingly magical place where you're working hard, but the bike feels chainless as you fly down the road.

That said, listening to music on the bike is a bit of a contentious issue. Some riders and coaches scorn it as dangerous (you can't hear cars) or even blasphemous (you should be tuning in to yourself, not Flo Rida). Others wouldn't dream of heading out without their iPod. Where you fall on that spectrum is personal. But regardless, you simply can't beat listening to music during indoor training sessions.

The real magic of music is that your nervous system seems to automatically sync with it. In one of the most recent studies to come out of Karageorghis's prolific lab, riders were told to pedal at a self-selected pace for a $\frac{1}{2}$-hour test while the technicians measured their overall work, distance covered, and cadence. The cyclists repeated the test two more times, while unbeknownst to them, the techs manipulated the music playing in the lab to speed up the tempo 10 percent and then slow it down 10 percent from the initial test. Speeding up the music program increased distance covered/unit time, power, and pedal cadence by 2.1 percent, 3.5 percent, and 0.7 percent, respectively; slowing the music caused those factors to drop off 3.8 percent, 9.8 percent, and 5.9 percent, respectively.

What's more, in two other recent studies, researchers found that listening to high-energy tunes not only increases your muscle velocity and force during explosive workouts but also helps you clear lactate and recover faster.

To make a playlist that will power up your pedal stroke, match the beats per minute of the music to the effort you hope to achieve. The chart on page 176 is a good guide. If you want to get really

FOR __ RIDES	CHOOSE MUSIC THAT'S __ BPM	BEST GENRE
Recovery	100–110	Country or hip-hop
Intervals	160+	Heavy metal
Tempo	140–150	Techno or rock
Endurance	120–130	Pop or alternative

scientific about it, you can download a free music analyzer app like the MixMeister BPM Analyzer, which will tell you the bpm of the songs in your library.

BELIEVE

All the brain training and mental tricks in the world will do you no good if you don't actually believe in yourself. Like the study of cyclists who were tricked into beating their personal bests shows, you have more in you than you think. No matter where you are right now, you can reach a little—maybe a lot—higher. Believe in yourself and let it out.

13

Get Fast!
Motivation

You'll get what you want faster when you know why you want it.

Fast Fact: Intrinsic motivation—that which comes from within—has been shown to produce greater task persistence, increased levels of enjoyment, and improved performance. Controlled motivation—that which comes from outside yourself—tends to elicit dropout and maladaptive psychological responses (like muscle tension). In other words: You have to want it for yourself.

—Adapted from L. K. Banting, J. A. Dimmock, and J. R. Grove,
"The Impact of Automatically Activated
Motivation on Exercise-Related Outcomes,"
from the *Journal of Sport and Exercise Psychology*

Forgive me while I state the obvious: You're not going to get faster unless you really want to. Seems like a no-brainer. Of course you want to. You're reading this book, right? Right. But do you want to get faster because *you* really *want* to or because you think you should want to? Or because you're sick of being dropped by the faster riders in your group? What motivates you can make the difference between turning up the watts and throwing in the towel.

The reason is simple: It takes a lot of work to train consistently and to train hard and to make the sacrifices sometimes necessary to do both. Unless you understand why you're training so damn hard in the first place, you can't reasonably expect to maintain momentum, says Charles Stuart Platkin, PhD, MPH, author of *Breaking the Pattern: The 5 Principles You Need to Remodel Your Life*. "Unless you understand the why of what you're doing, you won't do it very long," he says. "Just telling yourself 'I have to' is not a compelling reason to leave a warm bed to train first thing. Why is it important to you? What is your concrete reward?"

And let's face it, even when you know the why, motivation can still "ebb and flow like the tides," says clinical psychologist Howard Rankin, PhD, who draws an analogy to weight loss. "You go into your closet and find you can't fit in your favorite pants. At that moment, you're highly motivated. But you pull on another pair and go about your day, and motivation fades." In cycling terms, that's like getting shelled on your Saturday morning shop ride, but having a fun weekend and sort of forgetting all about it by Monday morning . . . until next Saturday.

If you've started and stalled out on your training more times than you care to count, waning motivation is most certainly to blame. But don't abandon hope yet. Where there's a will, there's a way. These strategies will help you figure out the big whys so you stay on track with all the training hows and whats.

SET GOALS . . . AND STEPPING-STONES

Without a concrete goal as your training anchor, you're a boat adrift and at the whim of the tides and blowing winds. You'll never get anywhere (let alone work hard to get there) if you don't know exactly where you're going.

Though this book is titled *Get Fast!,* I'll be honest and say that it's kind of a lousy goal in and of itself. Why? Because by itself it isn't definable. If you currently ride 10 mph, then 12 mph is fast. Or is it? Maybe you consider fast to be 20 mph. Or you don't even know your mph; you just want to be as fast as the men and women you ride with. Or you want to crack the top 10 at the local criterium this spring.

Take some time to think about what motivated you to buy this book. What did you see in your mind's eye? Now jot down those specifics and formulate a long-term goal based on those visions. The only rule is that it must be measurable. It can be based on mph: "I want to average 18 mph on the Pig Hollow loop by the end of the summer." Or it can be ride based: "By fall, I want to hang with the main Sunday morning group past Sprinter's Hill, where the ride always splits." Or race based: "I want to achieve a top-five finish in our local cyclocross series this season."

Some experts will tell you that goals shouldn't focus on winning. I'd agree that winning shouldn't be your sole goal, because you can't really control who shows up to any given race, and they may simply be faster. But if you want to win a certain race, you should absolutely state it as a goal.

Now that you have your big goal, add some stepping-stones— smaller goals that mark your progress en route to the big goal. It's like taking a trip to Miami Beach. You wouldn't just pull out of your driveway in Portland, Maine, without knowing how far the drive was or where you might stop along the way. You'd quit when you got to Pennsylvania and still didn't see the ocean.

Likewise, assign mini goals to every ride. Each time you roll out, have a plan for what you want to accomplish. If you're following one of the structured plans in Chapter 19, that should be fairly easy, as it is laid out for you in black and white. If not, make your own plan for hitting 3 major climbs, including 3 sets of 10 sprints, keeping your heart rate low for full recovery, or whatever you need to accomplish on that ride that will take you one step closer to your goal.

Finally, goals should be concrete and measurable, but not so rigid that they're unreasonable. Life happens. Unforeseen circumstances may sidetrack you. Or you may reach your goal more quickly than anticipated. Check in at the end of each month. Measure your progress and make any necessary adjustments.

Setting and achieving short-term goals greatly increases your chances for significant long-term success by building self-efficacy, says Jim Annesi, PhD, director of wellness advancement at the YMCA of Metro Atlanta. "Mastery experiences—being able to show yourself you can accomplish things—are most important," he says.

PLAN IT OUT

So you plan to ride "some time" Saturday. Then you get caught up sorting through the mail and organizing your tool drawer, and somehow the morning slips away. You make lunch with the full intention of riding right afterward, but your son informs you that he needs a ride to basketball practice, and before you know it, it's 4:30 and you have only 2 hours of daylight left. We've all been there. Don't be there. It goes nowhere.

Each week, sit down with your calendar, whether it's one hanging on the kitchen wall or sitting on your smartphone screen, and write down your rides. This will accomplish two goals right off the bat: (1) It will give gravity to your plans. When we mark something on our calendars, our mind registers it as a must-do and plans around it, which also makes it a nice anchor point for the rest of your day. (2) It gives your family a chance to plan around it, too. (Kindly share your plans with them if they don't have access to your calendar.)

Make following through on those plans as simple as possible by having your clothing, gear, and accessories ready to roll when you are. If you know it's going to get hot later in the week, have your sunscreen, water bottles, and lightweight jerseys good to go. If you have to go hunting for your gear every time you want to ride, there will be times when you don't.

FIND YOUR FLOCK

The single best way to motivate yourself to get out the door and on your bike to work hard and get fast is to find some fast friends to ride with. A fun group that meets regularly is nearly instant motivation. You know the time. You know the place. You know there'll be a bunch of people waiting for you and that you'll feel a million times better for having gone.

The right group will push you to ride harder, smarter, and better than you could on your own. A riding group will also provide some built-in checkpoints. You know the hierarchy of the pack within the first ride or two, who's the fastest and most experienced and how you stack up against them. Your goal is to work your way up the pecking order. And you will as you get stronger and more experienced yourself. No matter how experienced you are, there's a group out there that can put you to the test. It's just a matter of finding it.

You know you're in the right bunch when you find the ride challenging but not shattering (at least not every time). You should be able to complete the ride without getting shelled off the back every day (that's demotivating). You want a ride that is hard but satisfying.

Also plan to position yourself in the pack for maximum training effect. Often riders will position themselves toward the back with the hope of sitting in, which can backfire if the terrain is undulating. As you'll quickly notice, any time the pack hits a transition such as the start of a roller or an abrupt turn, there's an accordion effect, with the front of the pack slowing slightly, but generally maintaining their momentum. But the ripple effect of this slight deceleration is amplified as it travels through the bunch, especially when you hit the back, where you can find riders stalling out and then being forced to work twice as hard to catch back up to the front once through the transition.

If you don't have the legs or lungs to stay toward the front, keep your pace smooth by anticipating the slowdown and surge. You can always move to the outside of the group and pedal past those who are falling off the back, smoothly reinserting yourself into one of the many gaps in the pack that will inevitably form.

How often you should do group rides depends on many things, including your own personal motivation for riding with people. Most experts recommend doing no more than two, maybe three, hard group rides a week. If you simply love riding with people and find it easier to get out when it's with others, find another, easier ride to hop on for days when you need to roll easy and recover. Casual group rides are a fun, regenerative complement to the usual hammerfest.

CHANGE IT UP

Cyclists can be steadfast creatures of habit, taking the same routes over and over (and over and over) until they are shifting and pedaling on autopilot. That's not terribly conducive to getting faster, and it can be a little demotivating, especially when the weather isn't ideal.

When you just don't feel like going out, find something new to do. It can be as simple as doing your favorite routes backward (you'll be amazed at the new sights you'll see). If you have another bike, like a cyclocross bike or a mountain bike, take that out for a change. Maybe use Google Maps or another online map to build a ride around a brand new road. Keep your rides interesting and you'll continue to be motivated to ride.

You'll also see results faster, which always boosts motivation. Your body adapts to any given training stimulus relatively quickly. After a certain point, usually in just a few weeks, you hit a point of diminishing returns where that same workout brings less and less improvement. Variety keeps you evolving and progressing.

MONITOR YOUR MOODS

One of the first signs of overtraining is free-falling motivation. When you start getting stale, your legs feel heavy, fatigue is ever present, and you're usually pretty cranky about most everything. Jazzed to go out and hit it hard? Hardly.

Staleness is the end result of a string of biological disruptions such as rising stress hormones, dips in feel-good neurochemicals like serotonin, and muscle breakdown. The best way to avoid this state of dwindling enthusiasm and to stay fresh is to monitor your moods, says John Raglin, PhD, professor of kinesiology at Indiana University in Bloomington. He recommends "mood monitoring" to detect creeping staleness or overtraining before it becomes a full-blown problem. Like canaries in a coal mine, your moods are an early indication of when these biological factors are heading south. "With hard training, you're bound to feel tired and agitated. But that mood should improve with rest, and you should be ready to go by the next session. If your mood is persistently low, you need to pull back until you feel better. Overtraining is always a function of too little rest and too much training," says Raglin.

Take note, cyclists may be at a greater risk for getting stale than other athletes because they can literally ride themselves into the ground with little physical consequence. "Runners will break down physically with overuse injuries," says Raglin, "but cyclists can keep riding despite their heavy legs and exhaustion. You won't get faster by riding through persistent fatigue." Overtraining will rob all the joy from your rides. Plan regular rest and stay fresh.

SET UP A SOUNDTRACK

You read all about the performance-enhancing powers of music in Chapter 12. Well, the right playlist can also be highly motivating. I remember training for an Ironman a few years back and there were times—many times—when the last thing I felt like doing was going for a transition run (the run you do immediately after a ride). So I made a transition-run playlist and kept it cued up on my iPod. Those first few strains of my favorite songs ("Soldier Jane" by Beck was one such go-to tune) lifted my spirits and motivated me to get out the door.

Don't believe in riding with music? No problem. Cue up your get-started soundtrack while you're kitting up to get you in motion and put a motivating song in your head for the ride.

CONSIDER A COACH

Most recreational cyclists don't need a coach. But most could benefit from the experience of hiring one, if just for one season. For one, a coach will put together a tailor-made plan just for you. So instead of trying to come up with the workout of the day and second-guessing yourself, you have each day's workout all set up and waiting.

A coach will also help you set achievable goals, provide feedback on how you are progressing, and help you troubleshoot should you hit obstacles en route to those goals.

Maybe most important for some cyclists, a coach is someone to whom you are accountable. Having someone whom you have paid and who is working for you and checking in on your progress can be a powerful motivator to stick to your plan.

CELEBRATE YOURSELF

We all need a pat on the back now and then. Performance gains (especially if they land you on a podium) are a huge accolade in and of themselves; but let's face it, podium spots can be few and far between, and hard work deserves a reward.

Fortunately, there's no lack of potential rewards in this gear-centric sport of ours. So attach a few simple bonuses to your stepping-stone goals for extra incentive. Crack the top 10 in your local crit? Treat yourself to that speedy new set of wheels you've been eyeing. Didn't miss a single workout throughout the winter despite record snowfall? Consider a short bike vacation to somewhere warm. Or schedule a massage for every 4 weeks of hard work. It doesn't have to be expensive or elaborate. It just has to make you feel appreciated.

FIND YOUR FLOW

Whether you call it being in the zone or having a chainless day, achieving what psychologists call a flow state, where you are completely immersed in your ride, is what keeps us all coming back for more. For cyclists, this is when your abilities seem to be matched perfectly to the demands of the day. Riders often describe this state as "being one with the bike," like you're an extension of it (or it of you).

Obviously, you can't summon a flow state on demand (if only). However, you *can* take steps to help remove the barriers to your flow and to find and maintain that vaunted state of being—many of which you've now read about here.

To achieve flow, you need to feel adequately prepared, fully engaged, and appropriately stimulated by the challenge at hand without feeling stressed by it. In other words, the more you train, visualize, and practice stress-relieving techniques, the more easily you should find your flow. When you do, make note of the steps you took to get there. And most important, remember this is supposed to be fun. Keep your focus there and the rest will follow with greater ease.

14

Brain Care

Harnessing the power of your mind starts with taking care of your head.

> **Fast Fact:** Your brain lives on sugar alone. It burns about about 6 to 7 grams of sugar (the amount in two Hershey's Kisses) each hour just to keep you living and breathing. When brain glucose runs low, your levels of adenosine and serotonin rise, which causes fatigue, and your levels of dopamine drop, which interferes with your concentration. Mental fatigue can weaken muscle contractions up to 25 percent.

You mind is your most powerful training tool, helping you push through hard training blocks and willing you to carry on when every fiber of your being would really rather stop. It's important that you treat it right.

Aside from talking nicely to yourself and visualizing and all the brain training tips and tricks from Chapter 12, you also have to physically take care of your brain to keep it in optimum working order. Here's how.

SLEEP

Ideally, sleep is like a symphony. As night falls, levels of the sleep hormone melatonin rise, body temperature falls, and neurotransmitters such as serotonin and acetylcholine are released in a rhythmic manner that allows you to make the transition from being fully awake to drifting into sleep, where four stages await—stage 1, droopy eyelids, brain checking into slow, sleepy alpha waves; stage 2, light sleep as theta waves take over; stage 3, deep, slow delta-wave sleep; and finally, stage 4, REM, where your muscle tone goes limp and you enter dream sleep. You cycle through these stages every 90 minutes until morning.

It's during this time that your body recharges. Your body pumps out 80 percent of your human growth hormone (HGH) during deep sleep. HGH is a naturally occurring hormone that increases muscle mass and strengthens bones. This muscle-building elixir is released during the deepest levels of sleep—specifically, the ones you nix when you stay up too late, get up too early, or do both.

According to professional sports nutrition coach Donna Marlor, RD, CSSD, your brain's glycogen use also lessens by about 40 percent during deep sleep. Spend the night tossing and turning, and your brain will be sapping your liver's glycogen stores, leaving you more depleted the next day. And remember the stat above: A tired mind means tired muscles.

You already know you should try to go to bed at a reasonable hour and aim for a solid 7 to 8 hours of shut-eye a night (during hard training and racing, lots of riders push it to 9 or 10 . . . Heck, LeBron James famously sleeps half his life away, clocking 10 hours of z's a night). If that's a struggle for you, try to weed out these common sleep stealers.

LIGHT AND NOISE: Your brain likes it dark and quiet. Watching TV until the very last minute before bedtime can expose you to enough light to suppress your melatonin, and your body won't get the signal that it's time to drift into the first stage of sleep. Even that 3-inch smartphone emits more than 200 lumens, which is comparable to shining an LED flashlight in your face before trying to sleep. Shut off all the electronics about 30 minutes before bedtime. Try a dim reading light and a book instead. If outside light illuminates the room, invest in some blackout curtains to create a pitch-black snooze den.

Anyone who's ever been the victim of late-night partying neighbors or a dozen giggling girls at a slumber party knows it's tough to drift off when there's distracting noise. Nighttime noise also can disrupt your sleep—something I learned during a trip to a sleep lab for a story I was writing. I thought I always naturally woke up many times during the night. Turns out I'm just very sensitive to noise. So a passing train or even one of my snoring dogs could stir me awake. Since that trip, I invested in earplugs and have slept more soundly than ever before in my life.

BOOZE: A few too many drinks close to bedtime can wreck your sleep architecture. Alcohol consumed within an hour of bedtime lengthens your non-REM sleep and shortens your REM sleep during the first half of the night—so you stay in more wakeful stages longer. As your liver busily sops up and processes the ethanol from your bloodstream, your body goes into a bit of withdrawal. That creates restless sleep during the second half of the night, which explains why you feel so tired after a night of drinking, even if you went to bed at a reasonable hour. Turn off the tap two hours before bedtime.

CAFFEINE: Seems like a no-brainer, yet plenty of cyclists unwittingly wreak havoc on their sleep by pulling that last espresso of the day a little later than they should. Every time you use caffeine, it binds to your brain's nerve receptors, speeding them up. All that neuron activity fires off an emergency signal to your pituitary glands and you get a nice shot of adrenaline. That little buzz is all well and good when you're saddling up for a ride, but you don't want to still be buzzing when it's time to go to bed. The half-life of caffeine is about 6 hours, so even if your last java is at 4 p.m., by 10 p.m., you still have a shot of espresso's worth of caffeine flowing through your system, messing up your sleep and teeing up a vicious cycle.

TOP OFF YOUR TANK

Being well fueled at the start of a hard ride or race is paramount for optimum mental (and physical) functioning. In a 2005 study, South African researchers found that cyclists performing 1-hour time trial tests set their intensity levels during the first 120 seconds of the ride. Their selected intensities were directly proportionate to the levels of stored glycogen in their legs prior to the test. When they started the time trial carb-loaded, they paced themselves at a higher power output and sustained that output. When they started with fewer carb stores, they started equally strong, but their power output declined after just 60 seconds, long before they could have drained their stores. The central governor just started shutting them down early.

Keeping your tank topped as you ride will let you stay strong. Remember, your brain likes glucose. Bonking or even just running low on energy can cause a whole lot of mental distress. When your blood sugar drops, your perceived exercise goes way up. It also gets extremely difficult to keep the negative self-talk at bay, setting the stage for your central governor to pull the plug.

Marlor recommends training your gut to take in as many carbs as you can during races to stave off mental as well as physical fatigue. "Aim for sixty grams of carbohydrate per hour, up to eighty grams," she advises. Washing down some of those carbs with about

50 to 100 milligrams of caffeine will speed up the delivery of glucose into your bloodstream and fend off mental fatigue.

Remember to feed yourself off your bike as well. "Take in two to four grams of carbs per pound of body weight every day if you're training hard," says sports nutritionist Lisa Dorfman, RD, CSSD, a former pro triathlete and author of *The Vegetarian Sports Nutrition Guide*. "That's about three hundred grams from grains, beans, vegetables, fruits, and sports drinks for a 150-pound rider." Immediately after a hard ride, restuff your stores with 1 gram of carbs per pound.

STAY COOL

"Your brain has its own dashboard that monitors your body's fuel and exertion and temperature," says Carl Foster, PhD, a professor in the department of exercise and sports science at the University of Wisconsin–La Crosse. "The temperature gauge is most important," he continues. "When you approach overheating, your brain forces your muscles to slow down."

That's even more likely to happen when it's humid. Yes, it's a trite saying, but it's true. It's not just the heat, it's the humidity. Humidity sucks your strength fast, according to a recent study published in the *British Journal of Sports Medicine*. When researchers had cyclists pedal to exhaustion in a lab set to 86 degrees, then cranked up the humidity, the riders' performances plummeted as the humidity rose. The cyclists were able to crank along for 68 minutes when the humidity was a relatively arid 24 percent, but faded after just 46 minutes when the humidity reached 80 percent. They simply overheated as their core temperatures spiked.

Your best defense: precooling your core. Research shows consuming an icy drink (like a sports drink slushy) and putting ice-cold towels on your torso 30 minutes before go time can lower your core body temperature and improve performance by more than a minute in hot, humid conditions.

Once you're in motion, keep the fluids coming. Take in about 6 to 8 ounces (two to three gulps) every 15 minutes while you ride. Depending on your size, fitness level, and condition, plan on drinking about 20 to 60 ounces of a sodium-rich sports drink per hour. Remember you don't need to (nor should you) replace every last ounce you lose, just stay on top of your hydration. Use your thirst as your guide.

FEED YOUR HEAD

Training and racing can be as mentally exhausting as it is physically exhausting. Keep your brain in an energized, happy place by feeding your head—literally. We've established that your brain likes sugar. But it also thrives on healthy fat—specifically omega-3 fatty acids, which are essential for cooling inflammation in the body, managing your stress hormones, and even building brain cells.

Research shows that omega-3 fatty acids (found in salmon, sardines, and other fatty fish) promote the growth of brain cells in your hippocampus (the brain region associated with depression). What's more, hard training causes inflammation, which can reduce your production of the feel-good hormones serotonin and dopamine. Omega-3s cool inflammation, which could give your moods an added lift. Eat three servings of fatty fish each week.

Another high-test brain food: walnuts. Though all nuts are a good source of omega-3s, walnuts, which are particularly rich in alpha-linolenic acid (an essential omega-3 fatty acid), seem to deliver special health benefits. In a study at Pennsylvania State University, people who ate a diet rich in walnuts or walnut oil had lower resting blood pressure and less stress overall, likely because the fatty acids in walnuts have been shown to keep the stress hormones cortisol and adrenaline in check.

"Adding omega-3 fatty acids to your diet promotes vascular function," adds lead researcher Sheila West, PhD. That means you get plenty of nutrient-rich blood circulating around in your brain. Fourteen walnut halves pack 19 grams of good-for-you fats. Try toasting them for 10 minutes to make them especially delicious.

PART 5

FAST BIKE

How to spy (and buy) a speedy steed and turbo charge the one you own.

> Wider is faster. Rolling-resistance studies show that wider tires run at a lower pressure (gasp!), roll faster, and take less power to keep rolling than skinny tires pumped up to the triple digits.
>
> —Paraphrased from Lennard Zinn, longtime tech writer for *VeloNews*, based on the results from a study by the Wheel Energy testing laboratory in Finland

Cycling magazines, like the one I write for, have a rich tradition of gracing their covers with $5,000 to $10,000 bikes, praising their feathery weight and amazing speed. These pro-level bikes are known to be fast. And frankly, for a sticker price that approaches a down payment on a small home, they'd better be.

But you don't need to take out a second mortgage on your home for a fast bike. In fact, bike technology has come so far over the past 10 to 15 years that most tech editors will tell you that barring some box store special, it's difficult to buy a bad bike.

That said, you *can* buy a bit of easy speed by upgrading key components like your wheels, tires, handlebar, and maybe pedals and saddle depending on what you're currently running. You also can speed up your current ride without replacing a single part or component by performing proper, regular maintenance.

So rest assured, this section isn't going to be a buyer's guide of high-priced pedigree steeds. It's not going to be a new gear guide at all, really. Rather, the chapters that follow are a guide to getting the most mphs out of the bike you already have.

THE MECHANICS OF FAST

What makes a bike fast, anyway? We'll talk about how frame material, bike geometry, and general setup influence how quickly your bike accelerates and maintains its speed. *Spoiler alert:* Carbon isn't always the lightest or quickest material of choice. I picked up a friend's carbon race bike recently and would have guessed it to be a box store clunker if I'd been blindfolded. It was that heavy.

Bike maintenance and setup can also speed you up or slow you down. That gunked-up drivetrain increases friction, which can hamper your progress and hasten your fatigue as you need to generate more power to overcome it. It's also terrible for your components. As mentioned earlier, pumping those tires to 120 rpm may actually force you to produce more power to keep 'em rolling than if you let out a little air. In this section, you'll find the surprising (yet completely scientifically validated) reasons for this, along with other tips and tricks for maintaining your equipment—and increasing your miles per hour. As someone who once spent the better part of a 4-hour, butt-burying death march cursing her fitness when she actually had brake rub so bad that her rear wheel barely rotated more than a half-dozen times before stalling to a halt, I can attest that regular equipment checks can pay significant speed dividends. You'll find what to check, how to check it, and how often vital components should be replaced.

Finally, should you find yourself with a few bucks to spare on some speed, you'll find a list of the best upgrades for your money. You'll be pleasantly surprised how the simplest (and sometimes even cheapest) changes, like tires or even bar grips, can have a measurable and significant impact on your ability to get up to and maintain speed. The end result will be a fast, well-equipped (and well-maintained) bike that doesn't break the bank.

15

What Makes a Bike Fast?

Some bikes are simply built for speed. Here's why.

> **Fast Fact:** The lightest bike in the world (at press time, anyway) weighs just shy of 6 pounds—less than some wheelsets.

You don't have to go out and buy a new bike to get fast, but having a fast bike sure doesn't hurt, either. It's no secret that lighter bikes take less power to propel down the road, so they tend to be faster. But with the right geometry, heavier bikes can ride light and plenty fast. Remember, too, to consider where you ride. That heavy bike may not be such a problem in Kansas. Here are a few things to consider if you're in the market for a speedy new steed.

MATERIALS

One of the most important considerations is what the bike is made of. Generally speaking, there are four options: carbon fiber, aluminum, steel, and titanium. The material you choose depends largely on how much you have to spend, as well as personal preference.

CARBON FIBER: This nonmetal frame material continues to dominate the high-end bike landscape for a reason: It has many properties that lend to being fast. For one, it tends to be light. Carbon fiber is made of very thin strands of carbon that are coated with a stiff resin or plastic (which is why some riders jokingly call carbon frames "plastic bikes"). It's also infinitely moldable, so manufacturers can craft bikes from carbon fiber that are stiff where they need to be and flexible where they need to be. Plus, manufacturers can shape extremely aerodynamic carbon fiber tubes.

Carbon fiber absorbs road chatter, so the ride quality is smooth. A well-made carbon frame can be stiffer, stronger, and lighter than a frame of any other material. It's also the most expensive, and some still question the life span of a carbon bike. Though you should check the frame for cracks and wear as you would any bike, most frame builders guarantee carbon frames for life, as a testament to how durable the material is.

Also realize that not all carbon is created equal. You can find relatively cheap carbon bikes, but that low price tag buys lower-grade carbon, which is heavier, less stiff, and has a less responsive, dead-ride quality compared to high-grade carbon. If you can't afford a full carbon bike, look for one with carbon where it counts, as in the fork, which softens the ride.

ALUMINUM: I'll come right out and say it. I love aluminum. It's light, stiff, snappy, and lively. Most manufacturers have their own proprietary alloys, or aluminum blends, that include other elements such as magnesium, chromium, and titanium to name a few. Aluminum is less dense and lighter than steel, so manufacturers can make use of fat, beefy tubes with very thin walls, which stiffens up the frame without weighing it down. This stiffness equals speed when climbing and sprinting, but it can be a little harsh on rough roads, which is why a carbon fork is a good idea. Aluminum frames are also easily formed into aero shapes. Alloy bikes won't rust or corrode, but they can be damaged more easily than steel. Aluminum bikes tend to be relatively inexpensive, which is why you find many near (but not quite) top-of-the-line bikes made from this material.

STEEL: I'm resisting the urge to whip out the old "steel is real" cliché, mostly because I've never known exactly what that means. I imagine it's a nod to steel being a classic metal from the earth (mostly iron) and its being the material that the vast majority of

"Laterally Stiff, Vertically Compliant"

This is one of those phrases you'll read in a bike review, nod your head, and then think, "Huh? What the heck does that mean?" It means, simply, that the bike is stiff in ways that prevent a lot of side-to-side flexing, so your pedaling propels you forward without wasting energy while at the same time allowing some up-and-down flex to provide a little suspension and soften the ride.

Numerous features help make a bike laterally stiff and vertically compliant, including the shape and thickness of the tubes and stays, the carbon lay-up, and the size of the bottom bracket shell (that's why big, beefy bottom brackets are popular).

How do you know if your bike is laterally stiff yet vertically compliant? It will be comfy, yet quick to respond when you push on the pedals. Bikes that are too stiff will leave you feeling a bit beat up on long rides. Too much compliance makes the bike feel a bit sluggish.

bicycle frames throughout the world are made from. Because steel is dense, the frame tubing needs to be fairly slender. The thinner tubes flex more, and steel has a springy quality, so you get a smooth and comfortable, yet lively ride. Like any material, steel has some potential downsides. Low-end steel bikes can be quite heavy, and all steel is susceptible to rust and corrosion, so you need to take care to protect these bikes from rain and sweat. Some people contend that because they're less stiff, steel bikes may be slightly less responsive in race situations. But others say that difference is so slight as to be imperceptible. What's indisputable is if you take care of it properly, a steel bike will be strong enough to last a lifetime.

TITANIUM: This wonder metal was all the rage in the early '90s. Titanium falls between steel and aluminum on the density spectrum, so it can be used to forge a stiff, light frame that provides just enough flex to be supple. It doesn't rust or fatigue and it's darn near indestructible. One morning on our way to a ride, my friend's Litespeed mountain bike flew off a roof rack at 75 mph and cartwheeled down the highway, and all that broke was the aluminum seatpost. We stopped at a bike shop for a replacement and he rode the bike that same afternoon. The downside is cost. It's very difficult to cut and weld, so titanium frames are very expensive. Like other materials, low-end titanium bikes can also be heavy.

GEOMETRY

The geometry of a bike refers to the bike's dimensions and angles. Geometry has a profound influence on how a bike handles and rides as well as on how fast it will go at any given level of effort. Here is a basic primer of the key geometric components that can speed you up (or slow you down).

FRAME ANGLE: One of the key geometric characteristics that affects how any given bike responds when you turn the cranks is frame angle. Generally speaking, the more aggressive the angle, the more aggressive the ride.

Consider the head-tube angle. The head tube is the front tube on the frame, where the fork steerer passes through. Most bikes have head-tube angles that range between 71 and 74 degrees. The steeper (closer to 75 degrees) the angle, the quicker and more responsive the steering. A steep angle also brings you forward on the bike, more evenly distributing your weight between your arms and legs. Note that depending on other frame characteristics, this über-responsive steepness can make the bike feel nervous or twitchy. You won't necessarily ride faster if you're worried about wrecking. In that case, a more relaxed head angle (in the neighborhood of 71 degrees) might be preferable. Again, a slacker angle adds some stability that can translate into greater speed on the trail depending on the type of rider you are and the riding you do.

The seat tube is where the seatpost is inserted. The seat-tube angle affects power transfer when you pedal. Angles typically range between 72 and 74 degrees. Like head-tube angles, a steeper seat-tube angle means greater responsiveness and efficient power transfer. Very steep seat angles also give a rougher ride. So 73 degrees tends to be the sweet spot.

WHEELBASE: The measurement from hub to hub is the wheelbase. The longer the wheelbase, the more stable the bike rides in a straight line, but the less nimble it will be in turns. The shorter the wheelbase, the more maneuverable the bike.

CHAINSTAY LENGTH: Racing bikes are characterized by short chainstays, the bottom tubes of the rear triangle that run along the drivetrain. Shorter chainstays bring the rear wheel closer to the bottom bracket for a more responsive ride and better power transfer. Too short of a rear triangle, however, can make the bike twitchy and less stable than you might want.

BOTTOM BRACKET DROP: The bottom bracket drop is the distance the bottom bracket sits from an imaginary horizontal line between the front and rear dropouts. A lower bottom bracket drop lowers your center of gravity, which yields a more stable ride and helps the bike track better through turns. A higher bottom bracket drop allows more pedal clearance, however. So if you're racing crits where there's lots of cornering, you'll want less bottom bracket drop.

16

Maintenance That Makes a Difference

Proper care can make any bike quicker.

Fast Fact: To go fast as a cyclist, you have three main forces to overcome: gravity, air (wind), and friction. Proper bike maintenance can help you overcome all three.

I confess, I always feel terribly hypocritical writing bike maintenance chapters and features. I'm the worst about it. And I'm not just saying that in an "aw shucks, my bike has a little road splatter on it" kind of way. I truly suck when it comes to bike maintenance. I'm the queen of slapping lube on a filthy chain, bouncing my mountain bike on the driveway a few times to knock the chunks of dirt off, and generally neglecting my road, 'cross, and mountain bikes until they barely roll and then wondering why (well, not really).

I am not particularly proud of this. In fact, it's kind of embarrassing. So let's just say I'm perpetually working on being better about maintenance because I know, without a doubt, that when I work harder at keeping my bikes cleaned and tuned, I can work less hard at making them go fast. They just do.

Since I'm not a mechanic, and this isn't a book on bicycle maintenance and repair (although *Bicycling* magazine actually has an excellent book on that topic: *Bicycling Magazine's Complete Guide to Bicycle Maintenance and Repair for Road and Mountain Bikes*), this chapter is going to focus on the things that cyclists can (and should) do to keep their rides rolling at top speed.

THE STRONGEST LINK

A friend of mine once very wisely called the bike's drivetrain the kitchen and bathroom of the bike. "Even if the rest of your house is a mess, you want those areas clean and well maintained . . . just because."

Indeed.

The drivetrain—especially the chain itself—is what takes the watts you generate and turns them into forward motion. When this system is properly set up and maintained, its efficiency is astonishing. When engineers from Johns Hopkins University in Baltimore measured heat (wasted energy) generated by bicycle chains in a lab, they found that bicycle chain drives were up to 98.6 percent efficient. That means less than 2 percent of the power used to turn the front chainring was lost while being transferred to the rear cassette.

This is clearly a part of the bike you want to keep well maintained. The first order of business is lubricating the chain. It's essential, though maybe not for the reasons you'd imagine. Those same Johns Hopkins researchers tested three different types of chain lube—wax-based, synthetic oil, and dry-lithium-based spray lube—for chain efficiency. Guess what? There was not only zero meaningful difference between the products, but also the efficiency of a lubed chain was no better than that of a bone-dry one.

Now that was under spic-and-span laboratory conditions. Out on the road or on the dirt, you'd better believe lubrication makes a difference. Why? Because it keeps dirt out of your chain. The test engineers postulated that chain lubricant "is essentially a clean substance that fills up the spaces so that the dirt doesn't get into the critical portions of the chain where the parts are very tightly meshed." That's why you're supposed to clean your chain before you lube it.

To lube your chain, turn the bike upside down (or hang it from a stand or hook) and apply one drop of lube to the inside of each link as you slowly pedal backward. Once you've gone all the way around, continue backward pedaling at a faster speed for a few seconds to let the lube work its way into the chain rollers. Then take a rag and gently press it against the outside of the chain as you pedal to wipe off the excess lube (the lube is meant to be in your chain, not coating the outside, collecting grime). If you're using one of the self-cleaning lubes, you may need to apply a little more to saturate the chain so it can dissolve the gunk. Just follow the directions on the package. It's a good idea to lube your chain after every few rides, about once a week or so, and always after riding in the rain, since water washes away the lube.

The chain lube market is more saturated than a side of french fries. There are lubes made from oil, silicone, and wax, with a combination of ingredients. There are self-cleaning lubes (which means you don't wash the chain before applying), lubes you spray on, and lubes you drip on. Needless to say, it can be hard to know which one to choose. Your selection mostly depends on the conditions in which you ride as well as your personal preference. Generally speaking, you can divide lubes into three categories: dry, wet, and wax.

DRY LUBES: These go on wet, but set up mostly dry. Many contain synthetics like Teflon and run smoothly and hold up well. Dry lubes don't attract or absorb much dirt, which makes them particularly good for dusty or dry off-road conditions.

WET LUBES: As the name implies, these lubes go on wet and stay wet. They stand up well under rainy, wet conditions, but they do attract road dirt and grime, so you have to clean your chain a bit more often. Wet lubes are very durable, so they're a good choice if you ride on the road in mostly clean conditions.

SELF-CLEANING LUBES: These are wet-style lubes that lift the old lube and grime out from the chain and leave behind a clean coat. No separate cleaning is required. They tend to be durable and hold up well in wet conditions.

WAX LUBES: These lubricants dry to a thin layer of hard wax. They don't attract dust or dirt, so they keep your chain clean. Mountain bikers love them for that reason. There are self-cleaning wax lubes that are designed to allow a small amount of the wax to flake off when it comes in contact with dirt and grime, effectively keeping the chain clean. Wax lubes don't hold up very well under wet conditions, though, and aren't very durable in general, so you need to reapply them often, every other ride or so, depending on conditions.

How often you replace your chain depends on how well you've maintained it, how much you ride, and the conditions in which you ride. Replacing your chain once a year if you ride several times a week is a good rule of thumb. Some experts advise every 2,000 to 3,000 miles. Or you can periodically check the chain for elongation.

As your chain wears, it gets "chain stretch," which is bit of a mis-nomer for the elongation of the chain that occurs over time. What really happens is that the metal around the rivets in the links wears down, effectively lengthening the space between the links. You can use a chain-wear tool to check for elongation or just ballpark it with a ruler. On a new chain, there is a $\frac{1}{2}$-inch space from the center of one pin to the center of the next—or 12 inches for 24 pins. When those 24 links measure $12\frac{1}{8}$ inches, the chain has worn about 1 per-cent, and you could be damaging your cassette. It's best to replace your chain before it reaches that point. You'll be able to tell when the chain is getting worn because your shifting will be less precise and there will be more rattling in the drivetrain, both of which can slow you down.

PUMP THE RIGHT PSI

There are few maintenance factors that affect your rolling speed as profoundly as tire pressure. As I type this chapter, I keep flashing back to a 5-hour mountain bike ride over tough, technical terrain I did yesterday.

Because of an unusually dry spring, our trails are hard, dusty, and sketchy rather than their usual damp, tacky, and sometimes muddy. I inflated the tubeless tires on my 29er to the usual 28 psi (pounds per square inch) and rolled off with the group. (I tend to run a little higher pressure, a habit I need to break.) During the first 3 hours of the ride, I skidded out in corners a half-dozen times. Finally, after hitting the ground after washing out (*again*) in a tight turn, I stopped and let about 5 or 6 psi out of my rear tire. I didn't skid out again for the rest of the day. (This is why moun-tain bikers are constantly fussing with their tire pressure. It makes an enormous difference in bike handling depending on ter-rain and conditions.)

Conventional wisdom says that higher is faster when it comes to psi because more pressure means a smaller contact patch (how much of the tire touches the road) and less rolling resistance, hence higher, more effortless speed. But as the example above—as well as laboratory research—indicates, that's the case only on glass-smooth surfaces. And when's the last time you rode on one of those? Exactly.

You need your tire to be able to give a little so it can conform to the bumps and imperfections of the road, maintaining contact with the ground instead of vibrating and bouncing, which steals energy and speed.

Generally, narrow tires require higher pressure, and wider tires require lower pressure. On the road, proper psi ranges fall between 80 and 130 psi. Off road, those numbers are 22 to 45 psi. Instead of immediately pumping yours to the max, start in the middle. Then adjust according to how much you weigh and your riding conditions. Heavier riders should inflate to the higher ends of the ranges, lighter riders to the lower ends. On dry, hard surfaces, higher pressure will roll fast. When the road gets rough, losing 5 to 10 psi (say, going from 100 to 90 on the road or from 40 to 35 on the mountain) will allow you to maintain faster forward momentum. Likewise, wet conditions call for lower pressure for improved traction. On the other end of the spectrum, going too low puts you at risk for pinch flatting, where the tube gets pinched between the rim and a hard object like the edge of a pothole or a rock. So it's a matter of finding that sweet spot. I should note that tubeless tires are a game changer; I know guys who routinely push the limits and go sub-20 on the trails. This requires much trial and error to find what works best. But it's worth it because you can enjoy all the faster rolling benefits of low pressure without worrying about flatting. It's also a more comfortable ride.

As anyone who's ever let a bike sit idle knows, tires and tubes are minutely porous and air gradually seeps out. Temperature also affects pressure. Air expands when it's hot and contracts when it's cold. For every 10°F drop in the mercury, your psi drops about 2 percent. So it's worthwhile to check your tire pressure regularly, if not daily.

TIDY UP YOUR COCKPIT

Remember, the faster you go, the more power you need to produce to overcome wind resistance. That means all those loose ends start to add up against you—literally. The front of your bike meets the air first; so to fly fast, you want the tightly tuned cockpit of a jet fighter.

Check your handlebar. Are there cables shooting up like rabbit ear antennae? Do you have zip ties sticking out? Is your handlebar tape frayed? Tidy it up and flatten it down. Likewise, give a glance to the rest of your ride. Cinch down that saddlebag. Snip and cap frayed cables and/or those that are too long. You'll slice through the air more smoothly, which saves watts and improves speed.

WASH AND WATCH FOR WEAR

My friend Mike swears by washing his bike after every even slightly messy ride. He calls it "free mental speed" to have a clean bike. I can't claim to feel the same way. Quite the opposite, when I see my mud-splattered mountain bike, I remember the last great ride we did and feel like she's ready to roll right where we left off. But he does make the better argument in the great bike wash debate: The hands-on process of cleaning your bike gets you intimately aware of any important changes, such as cracks in the frame, loose bolts, frayed cables, or nonworking parts.

And in regards to those frayed cables and nonworking parts, brake and gear cables wear out and must be replaced periodically—

once a year isn't excessive if you ride regularly. Likewise, check your brake pads for position and wear. The wheels should be centered between the pads, with the pads slightly toed-in at the front. Most pads have a wear limit line embossed in them. When they reach that limit, replace them. On mountain bikes with disc brakes, you need to pull the pad to check for wear; if it's thinner than a dime, replace it. The shifting and braking precision of clean, new cables and brake pads delivers a smooth ride, especially at speed, when those things really count.

17

5 Fast Upgrades

Yes, as a matter of fact, you can buy speed.

Fast Fact: Wheels account for nearly 10 percent of the power required to propel your bike.

"What makes *that* bike so expensive?" I've heard the same question from readers, friends, and family members a million times. It's a reasonable inquiry. Very often you can find yourself staring at two bikes that are seemingly identical. Same frame. Same materials. Same color scheme, or "colorway," as they say in the industry. Yet the price tag can be hundreds, if not often thousands, of dollars more for one than the other. What sets that pricey bike apart from its less expensive counterpart? Components. Higher-quality components can turn an ordinary bike extraordinarily fast in a hurry.

As mentioned in Chapter 3, upgrading your wheels can make you 1 to 2 minutes faster over 40-K without expending a single watt more of energy. A good set of wheels can supercharge just about any bike. Believe it or not, so can tires. A few years ago, I was in the market for a new road bike. I tested a friend's sweet Independent Fabrication. The responsiveness was amazing. I was blown away by how it dove into corners with the merest flick of my hips. Then I tested another identical Independent Fabrication. It was still a stunningly great ride, but noticeably slower to respond. The difference was the tires. One had tubulars, the other clinchers. The difference in ride quality was night and day.

So in the spirit of making your bike as fast as we're making your body, here are five fast upgrades that will supercharge your ride.

TIRES

When you're on the hunt for get-fast upgrades, the first place you should look is rotating weight. Any part on your bike that you need to put in motion and keep going round and round uses the most energy and can significantly slow you down or speed you up depending upon how heavy or light it is. The most obvious rotating weight comes from your wheels. For cost and convenience sake, I recommend starting on the outside and working your way in. That is, change your tires and tubes first (lightweight inner tubes make a noticeable difference). Then consider your rims, spokes, and hubs (wheelset).

Like fine linens, tires can be judged by their thread count. And similar to those bedsheets, a higher thread count casing is the hallmark of a higher-quality tire. A higher thread count makes the tire lighter, more supple, and also more resistant to punctures. For road clinchers, the thread counts start at 60 threads per inch (tpi) and go up to 320 tpi for racing clinchers and tubular tires.

Tires also come in different widths, ranging anywhere from 18 to 28 millimeters. As mentioned in the opening to this section, don't be fooled into falling for the "skinnier is faster" philosophy. It's simply not true. Intensive head-to-head tests found that wider tires (28 mm) took nearly 5 fewer watts of energy to pedal 40 kilometers per hour than 25 mm tires, and about 6 watts fewer than 23 mm tires. The test engineers found that wider tires bulge less and therefore have less rolling friction than their skinny counterparts.

Tubular tires, on which the tires are sewn around the tube and glued to the rim, can offer the best of both worlds. They allow high inflation, but have low rolling resistance and are lighter than clinchers. The problem is they can be hard to change when you're on the road, and improperly glued tubulars (or ones that have been changed on the road and haven't had time to properly dry) can lead to accidents if the tire rolls off the rim.

On the mountain, you're more at the mercy of the terrain. There are a variety of tire widths to choose from, ranging from 1.8 to 3 inches (for serious hucking). For typical cross-country riding, 2 to 2.4 inches offers a lot of versatility without being cumbersome. Cross-country racers generally run tires that are right around 2 inches. The tread pattern should match your riding conditions.

Smaller knobs roll faster on smooth terrain. Taller knobs will help you get and keep a grip on rocky, rooty terrain. Wider tires are better suited to soft surfaces. For mucky conditions, opt for widely spaced, mud-shedding knobs and narrower tires. Of course, this being the real world, you're likely to find yourself on all kinds of terrain conditions, in which case, tires with tall, widely spaced knobs are a smart selection.

Both road and mountain bike tires are available in tubeless setup options. In my opinion, tubeless tires are a no-brainer for off-road riding. Though they're a little more work to set up, they are highly reliable, allow you to run lower pressure (no pinch flat worries), and vastly improve your bike's performance. Going tubeless on the road also shaves rolling weight and improves performance and handling, but unlike off road, where you can make just about any tire work, you need special tubeless tires that are designed with a specific tire bead that will not stretch and cause catastrophic blowouts at higher air pressures.

If you're going to spend more than you'd care to on any given upgrade, I would make it your tires. You'll feel and appreciate the difference immediately for a moderate splurge.

WHEELS

Because wheels are moving through the air as well as rotating, they provide an opportunity to fight two speed stealers: wind and gravity. There is a dizzying array of wheelsets to choose from. As this isn't a tech manual, I'm not going to even attempt to cover them here, but rather I'll provide some guidance to get you moving in the right direction.

First, look at the rims. From an aero perspective, box-shaped rims are your slowest shape. More aerodynamic rims will be deeper and "blade" shaped. The depth of rims varies from a few centimeters to a full-on disc with no spokes. Spokes are important, too. Common sense rules the day here. Round spokes are slower than blade-shaped spokes. More spokes (conventional wheels often have 32) disturb more air and are less aero, and thus slower than fewer spokes. Put together, the deeper the rim and the more bladed the spokes, the less drag on the wheel.

What's essential to remember, however, is that aerodynamics is not everything when it comes to wheels. You need to consider handling. Super-aero wheels aren't going to make you faster if you're weaving all over the road like a sailfish. Deep carbon rims catch the wind, often don't brake as smoothly or quickly, and can lack the rigidity that allows you to have confidence on rough roads, steep descents, and sharp turns. So before you go all aero, you might want to invest in a nice all-around wheel with a relatively shallow rim depth and lower spoke count that will provide decent aero benefits as well as stable handling in a variety of conditions.

The other factor to consider is weight. Generally speaking, you'll be choosing between carbon and aluminum. Carbon tends to be lighter, but also generally more expensive. Today's aluminum wheels are light and durable, and are often priced more affordably. Quality lightweight wheels come in at around 1,600 grams for a set.

Fast Accessories

Once you've upgraded your ride and are ready to rip, consider these final touches for getting fast.

Power meter: You've heard it a million and one times in this book alone, cycling is a power-to-weight sport. We've been working on making you stronger and lighter, so your wattage should be improving. A power meter will show you those results in black and white.

With a power meter, you know instantly how much work you're performing. Unlike heart-rate data, which is variable and affected by myriad factors including altitude, hydration, and temperature, watts are watts. Either you can produce the prescribed watts for a given workout or you can't. And when you can't, you're done. Time to rest. Power meters are also very good for literally metering out your efforts. If you tend to start out too fast and fade before the finish, a power meter will help you learn the wattage you can maintain for any given distance and dial that in. (Of course, that changes as you get more fit.)

Most power meters measure power either through a crank-mounted system or through a special hub. The downside: They're expensive. We're talking more than a grand once you buy all the bells and whistles you need. But for the serious cyclist, a power meter is the most highly

SADDLE

Stock bikes are often equipped with a heavy, middle-of-the-road saddle because manufacturers figure you'll be swapping it out for one you like better anyway.

Your best weight move would be to upgrade to a racing-style saddle. Racing saddles are designed to be slimmer to allow your working legs to go through their full range of movement in all riding positions without rubbing or chafing. The biggest weight savings generally come in the rails, with ultralight saddles sporting carbon

effective training tool money can buy.

Professional bike fit: Riding hurts sometimes, but it shouldn't be painful. If your back, knees, hips, feet, shoulders, neck, hands, or any other part hurts above and beyond the normal achiness after several hours in the saddle, something is amiss. A professional bike fitter will talk to you about your riding, watch and videotape you as you pedal, take measurements (often with high-tech lasers and cameras), put you through a series of flexibility tests, and in the end, make sure that your bike is set up to work with your biomechanics.

Aero lid: Any helmet will do for most rides and races. But if you're gunning for that local (state . . . national . . .) time trial (TT) record, an aero lid is the way to go. A good aerodynamic helmet can save 30 to 60 seconds for each hour of racing over a traditional road helmet. And you don't need to have a giant fairing running down your back to slice the wind. Bobtail helmets like those worn by Team Garmin-Barracuda and Team Sky are becoming increasingly popular among pro TT specialists. These aero lids look like a traditional TT helmet in the front, but the back is completely rounded off. That way, you can sit up, turn your head, and move about without negating the aerodynamic effects of your helmet.

fiber, which can shave as much as 30 grams off the weight of the saddle. (It's important to note that heavier riders are better off with sturdier rails. Check the weight limits when you buy.)

Even more important than weight is comfort. To go fast, you need to ride low and get aero. And if you can't ride on your drops without your sensitive tissues going numb, you won't stay there very long. Entire books have been written on finding the perfect bicycle seat (no, I'm not exaggerating). But I've got the basics of what you need to know.

Your weight should be supported on your sit bones on the rear of the saddle, *not* on the nose. The nose should help you control the bike with your thighs and support only some of your weight. Because of differences in pelvic structure, men's saddles tend to be a bit longer and narrower and women's saddles a bit shorter and wider. Some saddles also have channels or cutouts through the nose to help remove any unwanted pressure on sensitive tissues (this can also help shave weight). The best way to find the saddle that's right for you is to try a few through your local bike shop. The shop also might have a special memory foam pad used to measure the width of your sit bones to help pinpoint the right saddle width for your body shape.

PEDALS

Considering that your feet spin 90 revolutions per minute, 5,400 times an hour, and, therefore, tens of thousands of pedal strokes per ride, stepping up to a lighter pedal can add up to major weight (and watt) savings, especially over the long haul, since your legs will stay fresher (and thus faster) longer.

How much weight you can save depends on where you start, of course. But it's not unreasonable to expect to save between 150 and 200 grams—that's $\frac{1}{3}$ to nearly $\frac{1}{2}$ pound—by moving up to a high-quality, lightweight pedal. The lightest pedals on the market are generally made from titanium or a titanium/carbon blend. Don't use mountain bike pedals unless you're a mountain bike rider. It's wasted weight.

While you're at it, take a look at your shoes. Like pedals, lighter shoes mean faster feet. Top-end cycling shoes incorporate a lot of carbon into their construction for maximum stiffness throughout the sole and lightness everywhere else, which means more of every watt you produce transfers directly into powering you down the road as fast as possible.

High-end pedals and shoes can deliver quite a sticker shock, but they pay off. Engineers have figured that, because of the added effort required for moving your bike's rotating parts (like pedals), every 1 pound you add to your shoe/pedal system is the equivalent of nearly 2 pounds on your frame.

HANDLEBAR

You can shed some weight by upgrading your bar, but more important, you can dramatically improve your grip comfort and even bike control, making getting up to and holding speed easier.

Look for a bar made of alloy or carbon. One of the advantages of carbon bars is that they come in a wide variety of shapes and sizes, including ergonomic bars that are flattened in key places like the tops and under the levers on the drops so you can rest your palms more comfortably (some people find this less comfortable; it's a personal preference). Carbon bars are also better at absorbing road vibration, so you have less hand and arm fatigue on long rides over rough roads.

On a mountain bike, you'll want to consider your bar width. Many bikes come stock with a fairly narrow bar, which saves weight. If you primarily ride on tight, tree-strewn singletrack, stick to a narrow bar (so you fit through the trees); but a wider handlebar gives you more control, so it can improve your speed . . . and your confidence at speed. Grips are especially important if you ride rough terrain. You'll find different shapes, sizes, and materials. What's most important is that you can hold on and control the bike without beating up your hands.

PART 6

FAST TRAINING

Unleash your untapped watts and get fast—FAST!

Ride lots.

—Eddy Merckx on what aspiring riders need to do to succeed

Ever since Merckx uttered that now-fabled two-word mantra, cyclists throughout the years have branded it on their brains (if not their bodies). It's simple advice. And good advice . . . mostly. Unless you take it too literally.

Consider that the average pro cyclist trains 20 to 30 hours a week and logs 20,000 to 25,000 miles each year—farther than the average American drives in that time. That's what you call riding lots. It's also what you call being a professional cyclist. The rest of us are out there working 40+ hours a week. We have spouses and kids and all that comes with them. If we try tacking on another 20 hours a week on the bike, we are more likely to come to a grinding halt from utter fatigue than be flying down the road. The best results come from riding lots the right way.

Fast training for you and me means maximizing the time we have on the bike, while not sacrificing our enjoyment of it. I've seen far too many friends and friends of friends ride themselves into the ground and bury any joy they ever found in the sport along with the overtrained shell of themselves. The kicker? These same riders will lament about how they're tired and off the back and getting dropped before immediately following up the sentence with a statement about how they just have to train harder. Talk about missing the connection.

A LITTLE SUFFERING GOES A LONG WAY

All that is not to say that you don't need to work hard to be fast. You do. You need to suffer, too. Just in reasonable doses. So I've partnered with my longtime coconspirator James Herrera, founder of Performance Driven Coaching in Colorado Springs, to create a series of plans that will make you strong, fit, and fast without being worn down, losing your job, or getting kicked to the curb by your significant other.

You'll find Get Fast! plans for hill climbs, time trials, crits, and 'cross, as well as gran fondos and other fun rides. These plans pump up the intensity by focusing on short, sharp efforts on a variety of terrains. By gaining speed at shorter distances, you'll automatically increase your cruising speeds for longer rides.

To beat back boredom long term, you'll also find a section of all-time favorite intervals. After you progress through the plans, you can mix and match and create your own daily and weekly plans to keep the results coming.

REST WELL

All the riding in the world will do you no good if you don't rest. The hard riding you do breaks down your muscles, empties your fuel stores, and taxes your central nervous system. You reach deep inside yourself to squeeze out every bit of speed and performance, leaving your body spent. If you follow that up with more reaching and digging, you'll find yourself in a hole.

Instead, you should follow that overreaching with rest and recovery, so your body can repair and rebuild to be better and stronger than it was before. That way, the next time you dig and reach, you're starting from a faster, fitter place. Then you rest and recover and keep progressing in a stepwise fashion.

Recovery methods have come a long way in the past few years, and our understanding of how to get muscles mended and ready for action continues to expand as researchers focus their attention on this essential training element. You'll find out what foods to eat, clothes to wear, and other pro tricks for recovering right.

Finally, take a peek down the road and see what lies "beyond fast." You'll be surprised at all the places it can take you.

Fast Training Primer

All you need to know about teaching your body to pick up speed.

> **Fast Fact:** The average sedentary adult has a resting heart rate ranging from 60 to 100 beats per minute. A trained cyclist's heart thumps out a slow, steady 40 to 60 beats per minute at rest.

Technically, every time you saddle up you're "training," because with each turn of the pedals you're burning calories, strengthening your heart, and altering your metabolism. That's all going to yield what scientists would call a "training effect." In the beginning, those metabolic changes will also make you faster as your body adapts to the unique challenges of pedaling a bike. Once it gets the hang of riding, however, those adaptations come to a halt and you reach homeostasis . . . until you require your body to do a little more. That's where structured training comes in.

The difference between just riding around and structured training is that structured training is designed to create very specific fitness adaptations that will help you progress toward a goal—in this case, getting faster—more effectively. Speed training is strong medicine, however. So, though you'll make fast gains, it's important to understand how it works, how to meter out your efforts, and most important, how to recover adequately for it all to come together to keep you making forward progress without hitting the skids (i.e., overtraining).

THIS IS YOUR BODY ON SPEED

To understand how speed training works, let's take a quick look at what happens inside your body when you throw the hammer down. Consider your Sunday morning group ride. The pack heads out easy, and you're spinning in a comfy 60 percent heart-rate zone. At this exertion, your legs use mostly slow-twitch muscle fibers to turn the cranks. These fibers make the energy you need by taking stored carbohydrates, fats, and lactate and blasting them with oxygen in the mitochondria, the cell's furnace. Like windmills, this aerobic energy system creates steady, clean-burning power. The little bit of lactate you're producing is easily cleared and used for energy. The pedaling is painless; your legs are silent.

Now let's crank up the pace. As the pack starts to hammer, you jack up the intensity. Like overloaded fuses, your slow-twitch fibers start to blow. They scream for more oxygen to produce more power. You drop your jaw and start sucking wind. Your heart rate soars to 85 percent of its max to ship O_2 off to your pumping legs. Before too long, those endurance fibers need more oxygen than you can provide, so they call in the backup generators—your fast-twitch fibers.

These fibers make the ATP they need by going straight for your glycogen—or stored carbs—and blasting away without oxygen to produce lactate. This energy-producing system yields instant full-throttle power, but as with burning fossil fuels, it's messy work, dumping waste by-products into the environment. As lactate builds faster than you can clear and use it, you reach threshold. You've got 30 to 60 minutes at this exertion before the by-products of lactate metabolism create an acid bath in your muscle cells and you're forced to slow it down.

Speed training pushes your threshold higher, so you can ride harder, faster, and longer before the burn shuts you down. The biggest adaptation: improved oxygen use. Through a series of adaptations, you can increase the amount of oxygen-rich blood you pump out by about 32 ounces per minute while you're cruising down the road. You also increase your ability to use O_2 by the tune of about 10 percent for each minute you ride. In short, you can stay in your aerobic zone longer before hitting your threshold. Here's how it happens.

YOUR HEART PUMPS STRONGER. Like any other muscle, that fist-shaped organ in the middle of your chest gets stronger as you work it harder. When you push outside your comfort zone, you challenge your heart to deliver as much blood as it can to your working muscles. It adapts by getting stronger and more efficient, so it can squeeze out more blood with every beat. With more blood per beat, your heart rate lowers and it doesn't have to beat as fast or work as hard as you grind up steep hills, surge to close gaps, and sprint for the finish.

YOU GROW YOUR NETWORK. I saw Body Worlds (the exhibit where they have cadavers engaged in sports and activities to show the truly miraculous work of the human body) in Las Vegas a few years ago. I was wowed by the whole display, but the particular body that left the biggest impression was a cyclist standing upright. His legs had been stripped of everything but the capillaries, which had been shot full of bright red ink. It looked like a colony of spiders had thrown a rave. His legs were webbed solid with hundreds of thousands of tiny vessels to deliver blood to every inch of his quads, hamstrings, and calves. The harder you ride, the more oxygen-rich blood your legs need to produce energy. So your body forges thousands of new capillaries into your muscles to maximize your circulation.

YOU RECRUIT MUSCLE FIBER. You have two general types of muscle fibers: type I, which are your slow-twitch fibers, and type II, which are your fast-twitch fibers (and are further split into type IIa and type IIb). Your body is a very efficient machine that will use only as many muscle fibers as it needs to get a job done. As mentioned earlier, if you don't use muscle fibers, you lose the connection to them and they eventually shrivel up and die. That's bad. The good news is that you can keep them alive, well, and ready for action through regular speed intervals. Even better, though scientists used to think that our personal ratio of fast- to slow-twitch fibers was fixed, they now know it's a bit more fluid. So while it's true that some of us are born with proportionately more slow-twitch fibers and are better suited for endurance than speed, some of our fibers are switch-hitters that we can coax to behave more like one or the other depending on our training.

Some scientists have estimated that about 40 percent of the variance in our fiber type is due to environmental influences (e.g., training), while the rest is mostly genetically determined. So while you may or may not be a born speed machine, you have a lot of influence over how much you can maximize your power, speed, and sprint.

YOU IMPROVE EFFICIENCY. As you recruit and develop more muscle fibers, strengthen your heart, and lay down a thick network of capillaries, your body ramps up production of your aerobic enzymes so that you can extract more oxygen from your blood, and it expands the energy-generating mitochondria in your cells so they can hold more oxygen and make more energy more quickly.

MEASURING YOUR EFFORTS

If you're like most cyclists, you spend a lot of time riding comfortably hard. You know the place: just hard enough so you feel like you're doing something, but not so hard that you're really pushing it. That's an okay place to be sometimes. But spend too much time in this virtual no-man's-land and you risk becoming a one-speed wonder. To make measurable improvements, you need to spend some rides going slower to help build your endurance and some rides going faster and harder to increase your threshold and build speed. That means monitoring your intensity.

There are three common ways to gauge your workload at any given time: watts, via a power meter; heart rate, via a heart rate monitor; and self-perception, technically known as rate of perceived exertion (RPE), via how hard you're breathing. You can use any one or all three. Each plan has an exertion key at the top that explains the prescribed intensity in terms that work with your method of choice. Here's a snapshot of how each works.

RPE: The Breath Analyzer

Let's start with the least expensive, lowest-tech exertion monitoring alternative: your breathing. Since your muscles need more or less oxygen depending on how hard you're riding, the way you're breathing is a direct indication of how much work you're doing. In fact, nothing gives you as instant and honest an evaluation of your effort as your breathing does.

This method is best paired with rate of perceived exertion (RPE). On a scale of 1 to 10, how hard are you working? A 1 is coasting along a wide-open road with the wind at your back, barely pushing the pedals. A 10 is full throttle up a mountainside, legs afire, willing yourself not to vomit. Rate how hard you're riding by ranking your effort on a scale between the two extremes. Scientists devised RPE as a way to measure exercise intensity. Research shows it works just as well as a heart rate monitor or other equipment when you use it properly. The key is that you have to pay attention so you don't inadvertently allow yourself to push too hard or slack off for too long. That's why it works best in conjunction with monitoring your breathing. You don't stop breathing, so it's always there as a reminder to check your efforts.

James Herrera, founder of Performance Driven Coaching in Colorado Springs, created the training plans in Chapter 19. He recommends using the following breath-analyzer scale.

Zone 1: Light and relaxed breathing—barely above normal.

Zone 2: Deep, steady, relaxed breathing. That's your aerobic, endurance-training zone. It's an RPE of 3 or 4.

Zone 3: Slightly labored. This is a steady "tempo" pace, where you're working just a hair above your endurance comfort zone. It's where you'd be if you were riding with someone just slightly faster than you. It's an RPE of 5 or 6.

Zone 4: Short, quick rhythmic breathing. This is your lactate threshold zone, right where you're hitting your sustainable upper limits. Also known as race pace, it's an RPE of 7 or 8.

Zone 5: Hard, gasping-for-breath breathing. This is your VO_2-max training zone, or the top of your limits, as hard as you can go. It's an RPE of 9 or 10.

Heart Rate Monitoring: Follow Your Heart

As your effort ramps up, your heart rate increases. Monitoring your beats per minute with a heart rate monitor will tell you just how hard you're working. A few decades ago, heart rate monitoring was considered the gold standard for measuring exercise intensity. Power meters have now taken that top spot, especially among the pro ranks, but heart rate monitors remain a popular and affordable training tool. Heart rate is also another nice piece of information to have even if you are using a power meter.

If you've never used a heart rate monitor, it's a two-part device. The first part is a transmitter that sits on your breastbone right over your heart and is fixed there with a strap that wraps around your torso. The second part is a computer readout that acts as a cardio-vascular dashboard. You mount this computer to your handlebar (or wear it as a watch) and the sensor on your chest picks up the signal from your heart and transmits it to the computer so you can see how many beats your heart is thumping per minute. Most models also let you program your training zones and will beep at you if you fall below or push past your target zone.

If you invest in a heart rate monitor, you'll find instructions for setting your training zones based on your maximum heart rate (MHR), the highest number of beats your heart can pump out in 1 minute. Some manuals may still use the 220 minus your age formula (so if you're 40, your MHR is 180). Don't bother using it. Carl Foster, PhD, past president of the American College of Sports Medicine, has called the formula "useless," a sentiment that has been shared by many coaches throughout the years.

A better way to determine your MHR is to take a field test. That is, warm up thoroughly, then ride as hard as possible for 10 minutes, sprinting like you were going for gold for the final 30 seconds. Then cool down and check your monitor for MHR. Repeat this test two more times (with rest days in between) to find your true maximum. For the best results, prepare for the field test as you would a race. You should be well rested, well hydrated, and feeling good going into the tests. You should be breathing hard, but not panting uncontrollably.

Once you've determined your max, break your heart rate down into training zones to accomplish goals including endurance training, lactate threshold training, and recovery. Calculate your zones based on your MHR. For instance, a recovery heart rate for a rider with a 180 beats per minute (bpm) max would be <115 bpm (180 [MHR] x 0.64 [% of MHR] = 115). The following is how heart rate zones coincide with the breathing/RPE zones described above.

TRAINING ZONE	% MHR	RPE
ZONE 1 (recovery, easy day)	60–64	1–2
ZONE 2 (aerobic endurance)	65–74	3–4
ZONE 3 (high-level aerobic—"tempo")	75–84	5–6
ZONE 4 (lactate threshold—race pace)	85–94	7–8
ZONE 5 (max effort)	95–100	9–10

With all the formulas and numbers and percentages, heart rate monitoring looks like an exact science. It's not. There's a great deal of variation from one rider to the next. You may hit your lactate threshold (LT) at 75 percent, while more seasoned cyclists don't bump their LT ceiling until they reach 85 percent.

The human heart is also a little fickle. Your bpm can drift up or down depending on how many times you stopped at the coffee shop that day (caffeine, as you may have guessed, raises heart rate), whether it's cold or hot outside, and how late you stayed up the night before. Given its capricious nature, it's not always the perfect indicator of performance. For the best results, always pair heart rate with your breathing and RPE. It'll give you a more complete picture of what's going on.

Watching Watts: Power Meter Training

As you saw in Chapter 7, monitoring power gives you pure, instant, unadulterated feedback on how hard you're working. A rider can start pedaling and see that he or she is producing 200 watts without waiting for his or her heart rate to climb to a certain point. Power meters are extremely useful for training because they don't deceive you. With heart rate, you may be hitting 175 bpm, but maybe you're dehydrated or not well, so you're not actually producing that much power; you're just suffering at a slower speed. With power, either you're producing the prescribed amount of watts for your workout or you're not. If you're not, it's time to rest.

As with heart rate, training with power requires that you find your personal baseline numbers to work with. As mentioned in Chapter 7, functional threshold power, or the wattage you can produce for a 1-hour time trial, is one measurement coaches find most useful. Again, the way to determine that is by performing a 20-minute TT and multiplying that average wattage by 0.95, since your hour-long wattage would be about 5 percent lower, according to power training expert Hunter Allen.

When paired with a heart rate monitor, power meters allow you to experiment with cadence and gearing to find the sweet spot relative to your speed, wattage, and heart rate. Popular brands include SRM, CycleOps, Ergomo, SRAM/Quarq, and Polar. None come cheap, however. An entire setup still sets you back about $1,000. But for your investment, you get the most powerful training tool available.

TRAINING EFFORTS

Once you choose the tools you'll use to monitor your efforts, you need some efforts to monitor. The hallmark of training is working your body at varying intensities to accomplish specific fitness goals. That means intervals. By pushing your body outside of your comfort zone over and over, you get fitter faster as your body becomes accustomed to working at higher intensities.

As an example, let's say that when you start out you can ride your favorite 20-mile loop averaging about 15 to 16 mph. You incorporate intervals, where you ride several-minute bouts at 18 to 19 mph (with periods of recovery in between), and your body gradually adapts to the harder effort; soon you will be able to sustain it for the entire ride. You've effectively raised your cruising speed. Here are the types of intervals you'll be doing in the Get Fast! plans.

MAX: To raise your VO_2 max (the maximum amount of oxygen your body can use), you need to push your efforts to the max. These intervals are to be done full throttle, as hard as you can—Zone 5, or a 10 on the RPE scale. The good news: Because they're so hard, they're also very short, lasting 20 seconds to 3 minutes.

BRISK: If VO_2 max is your roof, lactate threshold—the point at which you start working anaerobically—is your drop ceiling. To get fast, you want to raise your LT so you have more aerobic room before you bump into that overhang. There are lots of ways to train LT, including climbing hills and sustained efforts. These efforts are done at an RPE of 7 or 8, or Zone 4.

STEADY: Also called tempo intervals, these efforts push you just above your comfort zone, so you're breathing faster and working harder than you would on a typical aerobic endurance ride. You're not working so hard, however, that you can't sustain it for a long period of time. Steady efforts improve your body's ability to clear and use lactic acid, so they also help raise your LT. They're done at an RPE of 5 or 6, or Zone 3.

CRUISING: Everyone loves a pleasure cruise. This is the intensity of a long Sunday ride. It's hard enough to feel like you're getting exercise, but you can carry on a conversation, cruise for hours, and enjoy the ride. These efforts build capillaries and endurance. Cruising rides are done at an RPE of 3 or 4, or Zone 2.

EASY: For hard intervals to work their magic, you need easy rides and rest periods to let your body heal, adapt, and get stronger and fitter. Your easy days and recovery periods between intervals should be ridiculously easy. Your only goal is to boost your circulation and promote repair and recovery. These rides hover in Zone 1, at 1 or 2 on the RPE scale.

RUNS: Did I just say runs? As in motoring down the road on your feet? Yep. There are these pesky barriers and run-ups in cyclocross races, so to get fast for them, you need to get fast on your feet, too.

PUTTING IT ALL TOGETHER

No matter what monitoring tool you choose, the following chart will help you work in the proper training zone. For your convenience, it's located in a key at the top of each plan.

PACE	OTHER TERMS	ZONE	RPE	BREATHING	% MHR	% FUNCTIONAL THRESHOLD POWER
Easy	Recovery	1	1–2	Light and relaxed	60–64	30–40
Cruising	Aerobic	2	3–4	Deep and steady	65–74	50–70
Steady	Tempo	3	5–6	Slightly labored	75–84	75–85
Brisk	Lactate threshold	4	7–8	Short and rhythmic	85–94	85–95
Max	VO_2	5	9–10	Rapid and heavy	95–100	100–130

FAST RECOVERY

Last, but very far from least, is recovery. There's an oft-repeated yet too infrequently heeded rule that you should rest as hard as you train, because that hard work will make you fast only if you allow your body to build back up to be ready for more. Remember, fresh legs are a cyclist's best friends . . . especially on race day.

You'll find plenty of rest and easy days in the Get Fast! plans. Take them. There also are techniques you can incorporate into your everyday riding and training life that will help you recover more quickly on a day-to-day and workout-to-workout basis. The following are some state-of-the-art as well as tried-and-true methods.

Water Immersion (e.g., Ice Bath; Cold-Hot Baths)

Marathoners swear by this technique, which is pretty difficult for this cold-water wimp to bear, though I have been known to sit in an ice-cold stream (along with dozens of other sun-cooked racers) after blistering hot stages of the Trans-Sylvania Mountain Bike Epic. Some studies find that immersing your legs in an ice bath for 5 to 15 minutes after hard cycling helps clear lactic acid and reduces inflammation, while others have found no such physical benefits.

Lactate levels aside, however, athletes in these studies do report feeling less fatigued and sore. In the case of performance, perception may be reality. In a recent study on water immersion, researchers found that, though lactate levels were unchanged, cyclists using cold-hot water immersion (a variation on the form in which you alternate back and forth for 10 to 15 minutes) for recovery improved their total work 14 percent more in repeated sprint performances than cyclists who just sat and rested.

It's not always the most convenient of recovery methods (unless you happen to have a spring-fed pond handy). But it's cheap, and may be worth trying if you feel like your legs take a long time to come around after hard days.

Compression Wear (e.g., High Socks/Tights)

Compression wear continues to be controversial. The International Cycling Union recently banned knee-high socks, seemingly to prevent racers from competing in compression socks. And the number of riders and racers you see wearing compression clothing is certainly on the rise. Yet scientists still can't quite agree if compression works.

Research suggests that compression tights can help reduce blood lactate levels and speed recovery. Studies also show athletes feel fresher and have less muscle soreness after wearing them. However, research linking these benefits to improved subsequent performance is still debatable. Recent, yet unpublished research from the Australian Institute of Sport found that riders were able to maintain their performance significantly better during 15-minute laboratory-monitored time trials when they wore recovery tights between trials. Most recently, researchers for the University of Calgary found that compression socks speed up the rate of muscle oxygenation during exercise, which could boost performance.

Personally, I'm a fan. I'll wear my tights while traveling to races (especially on a plane) and sleep in them during multiday stage races. They just make my legs feel lighter and fresher. I'm far from alone. At most big events, you'll find riders in the telltale high socks before and after their races (and sometimes during the race for some events). Unsure? Start with a pair of compression socks. They cost about 20 bucks and will give you a good sense of whether you feel any noticeable benefit.

Chocolate Milk (i.e., Moo Juice)

As detailed in Chapter 9, nutrition is a critical component of recovery. Sometimes it can be hard to eat after a grueling race. But chances are you finish thirsty, and chocolate milk usually goes down pretty easy when you're on empty. As mentioned earlier, it's also a quick and easy way to get some fast recovery nutrition. In a study of cyclists who rode until fully depleted, the pedalers who chugged chocolate milk afterward were able to hammer about 50 percent longer on their next ride before fatiguing than those who consumed a commercial carb-protein recovery drink. In 2011, two muscle biopsy studies on runners concluded that drinking 16 ounces of chocolate milk after a 45-minute run led to greater muscle repair and glycogen replacement than did rehydrating with the same amount of a carb-only sports drink. It's also cheap, convenient, and easy to toss in your bag. If you buy shelf-stable chocolate milk in the cartons, you don't even have to worry about refrigeration.

Foam Rollers

Foam rollers are one of those inventions I'm not sure how I lived without. Well, actually I do know how I lived without them—far more uncomfortably and with many more episodes of iliotibial band syndrome. I recommend a complete foam roller workout (see "Keep on Rolling" on page 70) to keep your muscles supple and knot free.

I've also found that if I use the roller soon after a hard ride or race, my legs recover more quickly and are less likely to get stiff and sore. There are many types of foam rollers to choose from, ranging in price from under $10 for a basic white roller to $50+ for more high-tech rollers such as the RumbleRoller, which is covered with 200 firm but flexible knobs that act like thumbs to dig in and knead your soft tissues.

Massage

My massage therapist, Rose, is my first stop when I'm tired, sore, and worked. Without fail, she leaves me with limber, pain-free muscles that are ready to go again. For anyone who has tried massage therapy unsuccessfully, I'd encourage you to ask for referrals and shop around. I'd seen about a half-dozen practitioners before finding the one that was just right for me. Not surprisingly, she's also the one that is just right for all my cycling friends.

What makes Rose so special is her myofascial-release techniques. My muscles and fascia get so many adhesions and knots that I get what I call pinball pain—a tight right glute pings down and leads to a twinged left knee, crosses over and gives me an achy right arch. She digs in there with her fingers, knuckles, and even elbows, releasing the fascia and separating all the muscles so they're in their proper positions and can work freely. It's amazing how well it works. I've had epicondylitis, iliotibial band pain, random hip pain, random knee pain, and dislocations of fingers, ribs, and shoulders. Through it all, Rose has kept me rolling along.

Up until this point, science has been stunningly slow to recognize the powers of recovery women like Rose have in their hands. Fortunately, research seems to be coming along. Early in 2012, researchers at McMaster University in Hamilton, Ontario, performed the first ever study that used muscle biopsy to look inside the muscle to see what was happening during massage. In the study, they had a group of cyclists ride 70 minutes to exhaustion. Massage therapists then performed a 10-minute massage on one of their legs, while the other leg just rested. When the researchers performed muscle biopsies on the cyclists' legs, the massaged legs had less inflammation. Even better, the researchers noted that massage signals muscle to build more mitochondria, which not only promote healing but also improve performance.

Space Boots

Along the lines of foam rollers and massage therapy are "space boots." Okay, they're not really space boots, but they sure look space-agey. These compression tools are zip-up leg sleeves that are attached to a generator. They have separate air chambers that fill in sequence, gradually compressing each muscle group from your feet to your hips, repeating for several cycles over a set period of time (usually 15 minutes) to stimulate circulation and healing.

The first time I heard of these devices was through Team Garmin-Barracuda (Team Garmin-Chipotle at the time), who were using a medical-grade compression device called the NormaTec MVP Recovery System. These devices work well, but they are *giant* and very expensive. More accessible commercial air compression pants are available through companies such as Podium Legs. I got my first peek at these during an early-season stage race in 2011. I liked them so much I took them home with me. They were a huge hit among all the racers in the bunkhouse. They're not cheap, but they are very portable and effective for making your legs feel fresh and ready to go after repeated hard efforts.

Fast Plans and Interval Mania

A little structure can yield a lot of speed.

Fast Fact: A group of cyclists who performed interval training twice a week for 6 weeks improved their 5-K cycling performance by 7 percent, according to a 2006 study from Ithaca College in New York.

For every goal, there should be a plan. By following a well-crafted plan, you ensure that you put in quality (not just quantity) time on the bike, working hard when you should on what you should and recovering and rebuilding right. A good plan makes sure you get fit, not fatigued, in your quest for fast. A plan takes the guesswork out of what you should do from day to day, leaving you with more energy to simply kit up and ride.

Following a structured plan is also motivating. You're less likely to blow off a ride if you have a specific workout on your calendar. By knowing your planned workouts well in advance, you can look ahead and make time for them. It also gives you a clear view of your progress as you look back and see how far you've come.

This chapter contains four plans crafted by James Herrera, founder of Performance Driven Coaching, to help you get fast for the types of riding most cyclists want to get fast for, specifically hill climbing, time-trialing, crits and cyclocross races, and century rides. In the Get Fast! spirit, these are relatively short, quick-hitting plans designed to maximize the efficiency of your training time so you can reach your goals without a huge time commitment. Each plan, aside from the one for hill climbing, is just 9 weeks long. The hill climbing plan is just 6 weeks long.

Following the plans is simple. Each day you'll see a calendar block with that day's workout instructions. You'll find the total time for your prescribed ride right at the top—in the below example, it's an hour. Within the rest of the box is that day's workout. The first line is the general pace of the ride (not including intervals). So in this example, you are doing a Cruising (or Zone 2) endurance-paced ride, plus intervals. The lines that follow are the intervals. In the ride below, you should include three 8-minute intervals at Steady (or Zone 3) effort with 5 minutes of rest between intervals (RBI). If no RBI is prescribed, allow yourself to fully recover at a lower intensity between efforts.

TUESDAY
1:00
Cruising w/
3 x 8 min Steady
5 min RBI

You will also find ramp intervals. As the name implies, ramp intervals start in one of the lower zones and work up to a higher zone over a period of minutes. These ramping intervals will develop specific pacing strategies for your event, allowing you to move from Steady to Brisk to Max pace as you near the top of your climb, completion of your sprint, or end of your race.

The block below includes a sample ramp interval. In this case, you have a 1½-hour ride at Cruising pace that includes three 12-minute ramp intervals: 5 minutes Steady, ramping to 5 minutes Brisk ramping to 2 minutes Max. Recover 10 minutes. Repeat 2 more times.

1:30
Cruising w/
3 x 12 min HC
(5 Steady, 5 Brisk, 2 Max)
10 min RBI

The best way to approach interval days is to warm up for 15 minutes and get to your Cruising pace. Perform the interval block. Then spend the remaining ride time at Cruising pace before cooling down for a few minutes. Pick your plan and let's get it started.

GET FAST!
Century Plan

The 100-miler is one of the holy grails of cycling. To pedal the century and do it well, we've designed a 9-week cycle that will boost your horsepower no matter what your current riding level.

Instead of burying you in volume, this plan is built on a medium-volume foundation, with block training (back-to-back hard days) and high-intensity intervals to accelerate fitness and speed development. By doing intervals on consecutive days rather than leaving a day of rest as you typically would, you achieve a greater training load. Though this is typically considered an advanced method of training, the 3-week loading cycle we've used here (2 weeks building, 1 week recovery) allows less seasoned athletes to safely push their limits and make fast performance gains without frying themselves. The intervals in this plan are focused on creating the strong, steady staying power you need for the long haul.

PACE	OTHER TERMS	ZONE	RPE	BREATHING	% MHR	% FUNCTIONAL THRESHOLD POWER
Easy	Recovery	1	1–2	Light and relaxed	60–64	30–40
Cruising	Aerobic	2	3–4	Deep and steady	65–74	50–70
Steady	Tempo	3	5–6	Slightly labored	75–84	75–85
Brisk	Lactate threshold	4	7–8	Short and rhythmic	85–94	85–95
Max	VO_2	5	9–10	Rapid and heavy	95–100	100–130

MON	TUES	WED	THURS	FRI	SAT	SUN
		Week 1 Total Time: 9:45				
Rest	**1:30**	**1:15**	**1:15**	**0:45**	**2:00**	**3:00**
	Cruising w/	Cruising w/	Cruising	Easy	Cruising w/	Event pace (aim for Steady) and terrain-specific; with group when possible
	3 x 12 min (4 Steady, 4 Brisk, 4 Steady)	5 x 5 min Brisk			3 x 15 min (5 Brisk, 5 Steady, 5 Brisk)	
	10 min RBI	3 min RBI			10 min RBI	
		Week 2 Total Time: 10:30				
Rest	**1:15**	**1:30**	**1:15**	**0:45**	**2:15**	**3:30**
	Cruising	Cruising w/	Cruising w/	Easy	Cruising w/	Event pace and terrain-specific; with group when possible
		4 x 8 min (3 Steady, 2 Max, 3 Steady)	2 x 8 min Steady 2 x 6 min Brisk		2 x 8 min best pace (aim for Brisk)	
		5 min RBI	5 min RBI		10 min RBI Record averages	
		Week 3 (rest week) **Total Time:6:15**				
Rest	**1:00**	**0:45**	**1:00**	Rest	**1:30**	**2:00**
	Cruising	Easy	Cruising		Cruising	Event pace
		Week 4 Total Time: 11:00				
Rest	**1:30**	**1:30**	**1:15**	**0:45**	**2:30**	**3:30**
	Cruising w/	Cruising w/	Cruising	Easy	Cruising w/	Event pace and terrain-specific; with group when possible
	3 x 15 min (5 Brisk, 5 Steady, 5 Brisk)	1 x 20 min Steady 2 x 6 min Brisk			2 x 10 min best pace	
	8 min RBI	5 min RBI			10 min RBI Record averages	

MON	TUES	WED	THURS	FRI	SAT	SUN
Week 5 Total Time: 12:00						
	1:15	**1:30**	**1:30**	**1:00**	**2:45**	**4:00**
Rest	Cruising	Cruising w/ 5 x 5 min Brisk	Cruising w/ 2 x 20 min Steady (1 min Max from 9 to 10 min and again from 19 to 20 min)	Easy	Cruising w/ 1 x 20 min best pace	Event pace and terrain-specific; with group when possible
		2 min RBI	10 min RBI		Record averages	
Week 6 (rest week) **Total Time: 8:15**						
	1:15	**0:45**	**1:15**	Rest	**2:00**	**2:00**
Rest	Cruising	Easy	Cruising		Cruising	Event pace
Week 7 Total Time: 12:45						
	1:45	**1:30**	**1:30**	**1:00**	**3:00**	**4:00**
Rest	Cruising w/ 3 x 20 min Steady (1 min Max at 7, 14, and 20 min)	Cruising w/ 5 x 6 min Brisk 3 min RBI	Cruising	Easy	Cruising w/ 2 x 15 min best pace	Event pace and terrain-specific; with group when possible
	10 min RBI				20 min RBI Record averages	
Week 8 Total Time: 11:00						
	1:30	**1:15**	**1:30**	**0:45**	**4:30**	**1:30**
Rest	Cruising	Cruising w/ 4 x 6 min (2 Steady, 2 Brisk, 2 Max)	Cruising	Easy	Event pace and terrain-specific; with group when possible	Cruising
		4 min RBI				
Week 9 (taper week) **Total Time: 3:00**						
	1:00	Rest	**1:00**	Rest	**1:00**	Event day
Rest	Cruising w/ 4 x 3 min Steady		Cruising w/ 4 x 3 min (2 Steady, 1 Brisk)		Cruising w/ 3 x 3 min (2 Steady, 1 Max)	
	5 min RBI		5 min RBI		5 min RBI	

GET FAST!
Crit and 'Cross Plan

Criteriums and cyclocross races are for those who love a little time in the pain cave. This plan is built on a low- to medium-volume foundation with an emphasis on building short, acceleratory bursts of power, to give you the legs you need to repeatedly surge and recover over a 1- to 2-hour time frame. This 9-week plan uses a 3-week loading cycle, including three high-intensity rides followed by a day of recovery each week. This training structure allows you to build maximum power without overtaxing your system. For the cyclocross (CX) riders in the crowd, you'll also find specific supplemental workouts that include short runs, sprints, and skill development.

PACE	OTHER TERMS	ZONE	RPE	BREATHING	% MHR	% FUNCTIONAL THRESHOLD POWER
Easy	Recovery	1	1–2	Light and relaxed	60–64	30–40
Cruising	Aerobic	2	3–4	Deep and steady	65–74	50–70
Steady	Tempo	3	5–6	Slightly labored	75–84	75–85
Brisk	Lactate threshold	4	7–8	Short and rhythmic	85–94	85–95
Max	VO_2	5	9–10	Rapid and heavy	95–100	100–130

MON	TUES	WED	THURS	FRI	SAT	SUN

Week 1 Total Time: 7:15

MON	TUES	WED	THURS	FRI	SAT	SUN
	1:00	1:00	1:00	0:45	2:00	1:30
Rest	Cruising w/ 4 x 6 min (2 Steady, 2 Brisk, 2 Steady)	Cruising w/ skill practice (e.g., cornering and accelerating out of corners; CX specifics: run-ups, dismount/ mount)	Cruising w/ 3 x 8 min (2 Brisk, 2 Steady, 2 Brisk, 2 Steady)	Easy	Cruising w/ 30 min CX- or crit-specific course riding	Cruising
	4 min RBI		5 min RBI		CX: 5 x 40 m run sprints	

Week 2 Total Time: 8:15

MON	TUES	WED	THURS	FRI	SAT	SUN
	1:15	1:00	1:30	0:45	2:15	1:30
Rest	Cruising w/ 5 x 6 min (2 Steady, 2 Brisk, 2 Steady)	Cruising w/ skill practice (e.g., cornering and accelerating out of corners; CX specifics: run-ups, dismount/ mount)	Cruising w/ 3 x 10 min (2 Brisk, 2 Steady, 2 Brisk, 2 Steady, 2 Brisk)	Easy	Cruising w/ 30 min CX- or crit-specific course riding CX: 6 x 20 m uphill run sprints	Cruising
	3 min RBI	CX: 20 min Steady	8 min RBI			

Week 3 (rest week) **Total Time: 6:15**

MON	TUES	WED	THURS	FRI	SAT	SUN
	1:00	1:00	1:00	0:45	1:30	1:00
Rest	Cruising	Easy w/ skill practice (e.g., cornering and accelerating out of corners; CX specifics: run-ups, dismount/ mount)	Cruising	Easy	Cruising w/ 30 min CX- or crit-specific course riding	Cruising
		CX: 15 min Steady			CX: 15 min Steady	

MON	TUES	WED	THURS	FRI	SAT	SUN
Week 4 Total Time: 8:30						
	1:30	**1:00**	**1:30**	**0:45**	**2:15**	**1:30**
Rest	Cruising w/ 5 x 6 min (2 Steady, 1 Max, 2 Steady, 1 Max)	Cruising w/ skill practice (e.g., cornering and accelerating out of corners; CX specifics: run-ups, dismount/ mount)	Cruising w/ 3 x 12 min: (alternate 1 Max, 3 Steady x 3)	Easy	Cruising w/ 45 min CX- or crit-specific course riding	Cruising
	4 min RBI	CX: 20 min Steady	6 min RBI		CX: 8 x 40 m run sprints	
Week 5 Total Time: 8:45						
	1:30	**1:00**	**1:30**	**0:45**	**2:30**	**1:30**
Rest	Cruising w/ 4 x 8 min (2 Steady, 2 Max, 2 Steady, 2 Max)	Cruising w/ skill practice (e.g., cornering and accelerating out of corners; CX specifics: run-ups, dismount/ mount)	Cruising w/ 3 x 12 min: (alternate 2 Max, 2 Steady x 3)	Easy	Cruising w/ 45 min CX- or crit-specific course riding	Cruising
	4 min RBI	CX: 20 min Steady	6 min RBI		CX: 8 x 20 m uphill run sprints	
Week 6 (rest week) **Total Time: 6:45**						
	1:00	**1:00**	**1:00**	**0:45**	**1:30**	**1:30**
Rest	Cruising	Easy w/ skill practice (e.g., cornering and accelerating out of corners; CX specifics: run-ups, dismount/ mount)	Cruising	Easy	Cruising w/ 30 min CX- or crit-specific course riding	Cruising
		CX: 15 min Steady			CX: 15 min Steady	

MON	TUES	WED	THURS	FRI	SAT	SUN
Week 7 Total Time: 8:15						
	1:30	**1:00**	**1:30**	**0:45**	**2:00**	**1:30**
Rest	Cruising w/	Cruising w/	Cruising w/	Easy		Cruising
	4 x 10 min (3 Max, 2 Steady, 3 Max, 2 Steady)	skill practice (e.g., cornering and accelerating out of corners; CX specifics: run-ups, dismount/mount)	1 x 6 min Steady 4 x 90 sec RBI		CX- or crit-specific course riding 70% of race time	
	6 min RBI	CX: 20 min Steady	4 min RBI			
Week 8 Total Time: 7:15						
	1:15	**1:00**	**1:15**	**0:45**	**1:45**	**1:15**
Rest	Cruising w/	Cruising w/	Cruising	Easy	Cruising w/	Cruising
	2 x 10 min Steady	skill practice (e.g., cornering and accelerating out of corners; CX specifics: run-ups, dismount/mount)	1 x 10 min Steady 4 x 3 min Max		30 min CX- or crit-specific course riding	
	6 min RBI	CX: 15 min Steady	3 min RBI		CX: 4 x 40 m run sprints	
Week 9 (taper week) **Total Time: 4:45**						
	1:00	**1:00**	**1:00**	**0:45**	**1:00**	**1:00**
Rest	Cruising w/	Rest	Cruising w/	Easy	Cruising w/	Cruising w/
	1 x 8 min Steady 5 x 90 sec Max		1 x 5 min Steady 4 x 90 sec Max		30 min CX- or crit-specific course riding 4 x 1 min Max	CX- or crit-specific course riding
	4 min RBI		4 min RBI		5 min RBI	

GET FAST!
Time Trial Plan

With big overloads come big adaptations. Our low- to mid-volume time trial (TT) plan focuses on the high-intensity demands of the race against the clock. The 3-week loading cycle includes a mix of Steady and Brisk efforts with short recoveries, plus time trial specific work. This will give you the opportunity to improve your time at TT intensity while also adjusting and growing accustomed to your bike and positioning. Whether you race your local time trials, compete in triathlons, or just want to kick a little tail in a club ride, this plan will give you the speed you need.

PACE	OTHER TERMS	ZONE	RPE	BREATHING	% MHR	% FUNCTIONAL THRESHOLD POWER
Easy	Recovery	1	1–2	Light and relaxed	60–64	30–40
Cruising	Aerobic	2	3–4	Deep and steady	65–74	50–70
Steady	Tempo	3	5–6	Slightly labored	75–84	75–85
Brisk	Lactate threshold	4	7–8	Short and rhythmic	85–94	85–95
Max	VO$_2$	5	9–10	Rapid and heavy	95–100	100–130

MON	TUES	WED	THURS	FRI	SAT	SUN
Week 1 Total Time: 7:30						
	1:00	**1:15**	**1:00**	**0:45**	**2:00**	**1:30**
Rest	Cruising w/	Cruising	Cruising w/	Easy	Cruising w/	Cruising
	1 x 12 min Steady 4 x 5 min Brisk		1 x 10 min Steady 4 x 5 min Brisk		3 x 10 min TT	
	3 min RBI		3 min RBI		8 min RBI	
Week 2 Total Time: 8:15						
	1:15	**1:00**	**1:15**	**0:45**	**2:30**	**1:30**
Rest	Cruising w/	Cruising	Cruising w/	Easy	Cruising w/	Cruising
	1 x 10 min Steady 5 x 5 min Brisk		3 x 10 min (2 Steady, 8 Brisk)		2 x 15 min TT	
	3 min RBI		5 min RBI		8 min RBI	
Week 3 (rest week) **Total Time: 5:45**						
	1:00	**0:45**	**1:00**		**1:45**	**1:15**
Rest	Cruising	Easy	Cruising	Rest	Cruising	Cruising
Week 4 Total Time: 8:30						
	1:30	**1:00**	**1:15**	**1:00**	**2:15**	**1:30**
Rest	Cruising w/	Cruising	Cruising w/	Easy	Cruising w/	Cruising
	1 x 10 min Steady 6 x 2 min Max		3 x 12 min (2 Steady, 10 Brisk)		3 x 12 min TT	
	3 min RBI		6 min RBI		6 min RBI	
Week 5 Total Time: 9:15						
	1:30	**1:00**	**1:30**	**1:00**	**2:30**	**1:45**
Rest	Cruising w/	Cruising	Cruising w/	Easy	Cruising w/	Cruising
	1 x 10 min Steady 5 x 3 min Max		3 x 15 min (3 Steady, 12 Brisk)		2 x 20 min TT	
	2 min RBI		8 min RBI		8 min RBI	

MON	TUES	WED	THURS	FRI	SAT	SUN
Week 6 (rest week) **Total Time: 6:45**						
	1:00	**0:45**	**1:00**	**0:45**	**2:00**	**1:15**
Rest	Cruising	Easy	Cruising	Easy	Cruising	Cruising
Week 7 Total Time: 8:45						
	1:30	**1:00**	**1:30**	**1:00**	**2:00**	**1:45**
Rest	Cruising w/ 1 x 10 min Steady 4 x 4 min Max 2 min RBI	Cruising	Cruising w/ 1 x 10 min Steady 5 x 2 min Max 2 min RBI	Easy	1 x 45 min TT	Cruising
Week 8 Total Time: 8:00						
	1:30	**1:00**	**1:30**	**1:00**	**1:45**	**1:15**
Rest	Cruising w/ 2 x 15 min Steady 10 min RBI	Cruising	Cruising w/ 5 x 4 min Max 2 min RBI	Easy	Cruising w/ 2 x 6 min TT 10 min RBI	Cruising
Week 9 (taper week) **Total Time: 3:45**						
	1:00		**1:00**	**0:45**	**1:00**	
Rest	Cruising w/ 4 x 5 min (2 Steady, 2 Brisk, 1 Max) 5 min RBI	Rest	Cruising w/ 4 x 4 min (2 Steady, 2 Brisk) 5 min RBI	Easy	Cruising w/ 4 x 1 min Max 5 min RBI	40-K TT

GET FAST!
Hill Climb Plan

This 6-week plan is designed to push your hill climbing (HC) abilities over the top in a relatively short period of time. We used a mid-volume approach with plenty of block- and single-day loading strategies to keep the intensity high and the adaptations coming.

PACE	OTHER TERMS	ZONE	RPE	BREATHING	% MHR	% FUNCTIONAL THRESHOLD POWER
Easy	Recovery	1	1–2	Light and relaxed	60–64	30–40
Cruising	Aerobic	2	3–4	Deep and steady	65–74	50–70
Steady	Tempo	3	5–6	Slightly labored	75–84	75–85
Brisk	Lactate threshold	4	7–8	Short and rhythmic	85–94	85–95
Max	VO$_2$	5	9–10	Rapid and heavy	95–100	100–130

MON	TUES	WED	THURS	FRI	SAT	SUN
	Week 1 Total Time: 8:15					
	1:30	**1:30**	**1:00**	**0:45**	**2:00**	**1:30**
Rest	Cruising w/ 3 x 15 min Steady HC 8–10 min RBI	Cruising w/ 5 x 6 min Brisk HC 4–5 min RBI	Cruising	Easy	Cruising w/ 3 x 10 min HC (5 Steady, 5 Brisk) RBI on descent	Cruising
	Week 2 Total Time: 9:00					
	1:30	**1:00**	**1:30**	**1:00**	**2:15**	**1:45**
Rest	Cruising w/ 3 x 12 min HC (5 Steady, 5 Brisk, 2 Max) 10 min RBI	Cruising	Cruising w/ 4 x 8 min Brisk HC RBI on descent	Easy	Cruising w/ 3 x 15 min HC (5 Steady, 8 Brisk, 2 Max) 10 min RBI	Cruising
	Week 3 (rest week) **Total Time: 6:00**					
	1:00		**1:00**	**0:45**	**2:00**	**1:15**
Rest	Cruising	Rest	Cruising	Easy	Cruising 1 x 10 min Steady HC	Cruising
	Week 4 Total Time: 9:30					
	1:30	**1:30**	**1:00**	**1:00**	**2:30**	**2:00**
Rest	Cruising w/ 2 x 20 min HC (5 Steady, 12 Brisk, 3 Max) 10 min RBI	Cruising w/ 4 x 6 min Brisk HC 4–5 min RBI	Cruising	Easy	HC simulation course or time- and grade-specific course	Cruising

MON	TUES	WED	THURS	FRI	SAT	SUN
			Week 5 Total Time: 8:30			
	1:00	**1:45**	**1:15**	**1:00**	**2:00**	**1:30**
Rest	Cruising	Cruising w/ 1 x 30 min HC (5 Steady, 22 Brisk, 3 Max)	Cruising	Easy	Cruising w/ 3 x 6 min Brisk HC	Cruising
					RBI on descent	
			Week 6 (taper week) **Total Time: 5:15**			
	1:30		**1:00**	**0:45**	**1:00**	**1:00**
Rest	Cruising w/ 4 x 4 min Brisk HC	Rest	Cruising w/ 3 x 5 min HC (2 Steady, 2 Brisk, 1 Max)	Easy	Cruising w/ 4 x 3 min (1 Steady, 1 Brisk, 1 Max)	HC
	5 min RBI		8 min RBI		5 min RBI	

INTERVAL MANIA

Whether or not you choose to follow one of the specific training plans, you should definitely do interval training if you want to get fast. Don't groan. These quick, sometimes eye-popping efforts may induce misery in the short term, but they offer huge fitness returns for a comparatively small time investment. Even 20- to 30-second microintervals have been shown to increase VO_2 max, burn fat, build muscle, and even improve endurance. And they work fast. In a study of 38 conditioned cyclists, Australian researchers found that those doing high-intensity interval training twice a week slashed their 40-K time trial time by nearly 3 minutes (about 5 percent) and improved their average speed by nearly 1 mph.

"We know even highly trained riders can increase their stroke volume [how much blood the heart pumps per beat], increase the delivery of oxygen and nutrients to muscles, and improve the muscles' ability to extract oxygen," says study author and exercise physiologist Paul Laursen, PhD. Intervals also seem to make your powerful, sprint-happy fast-twitch fibers more fatigue resistant, so they behave more like slow-twitch fibers; then you can go really fast for longer. "Just two weeks of training can enhance performance," says Laursen.

The following are intervals to match all your Get Fast! needs. If you're not following a plan or you want to get creative and make your own, add one or more of the following interval workouts to your rides twice a week. Always warm up with easy pedaling for at least 15 minutes. Cool down as needed.

Muscular Endurance

Build power and train your body to recover quickly between efforts for events that demand repeated surges.

40/20s: In a medium to large gear, push hard for 40 seconds. Recover for 20 seconds. Repeat 10 times. That's 1 set. Do up to 4, resting 5 minutes between sets.

30-second blasts: In a medium to large gear, sprint all out for 30 seconds, then spin easy for $2\frac{1}{2}$ minutes. Do this 12 times. Spin easy to cool down.

Sprinting Speed

These lightning-fast efforts help you develop a fluid and efficient cadence, as well as sheer speed.

Flying finishes: At the end of a long ride, shift to a big gear and sprint 100 percent for 30 seconds. Rest for 15 seconds. Repeat 8 to 10 times. Recover completely. Repeat for another set. Keep the effort consistent during each interval.

High-speed spin-ups: On a flat road (or on the trainer with low resistance), spin a very high cadence (approximately 120 rpm) for 5 to 10 minutes. Work up (about 5 minutes at a time) to spinning a rapid cadence for 30 minutes.

Climb Stronger

Develop your climbing power, prowess, and style with these targeted efforts.

Hill charge: On a moderate incline, stand out of the saddle and charge up the hill as fast as possible for 30 seconds. Coast back to your starting point. Repeat, this time seated. Alternate between standing and sitting for 6 climbs. Recover 10 minutes. Do another set.

Gear jammer: On a long, moderate climb, start climbing at an 80 to 85 rpm cadence. Click down to the next hardest gear and try to maintain your cadence for 2 minutes. Shift back to an easier gear and recover for 2 minutes. Repeat the climb.

Build Power

Strength plus speed equals power. Here are drills to get both.

Tabata intervals: In a moderate to hard gear, sprint as hard as possible for 20 seconds. Coast for 10 seconds. Repeat 6 to 8 times. Do 3 sets.

Monster gear push: Click into a harder gear or start up a hill incline until you are pedaling against a resistance that slows your cadence to about 55 to 65 rpm. Concentrate on keeping your pedal stroke smooth and circular. Push for 5 minutes. Recover for $2\frac{1}{2}$ minutes (half the interval time). Repeat 2 to 3 times. Gradually work your way up to 10-minute intervals done 4 or 5 times, with 5 minutes of recovery in between. Skip these if you have a history of knee problems.

Increase Your Threshold

Raising your threshold pace will help you sustain attacks.

Bridging the gap: Ride as hard as you can for 2 to 3 minutes, as though you are chasing down a rider that's attacking (you should be flagging by the end). Recover at an easy pace for 1 to 2 minutes. Do up to 3 sets.

Lactate threshold climbing surges: Find a moderate hill you can climb seated while maintaining a cadence of about 80 rpm. Staying seated, surge until you're just above your lactate threshold for 1 minute. Recover for 2 minutes. Repeat all the way up the climb, or for about 10 to 15 minutes.

20

Beyond Fast

For every thing there is a season.
—Ecclesiastes 3:1

I've been watching my friend and teammate Cheryl work her way into a breakthrough year this season. She spent the winter with laser focus, working with a coach, performing base miles and specific, targeted timed intervals. She visualized, cleaned up her diet, strengthened and stretched, and schooled herself with books on mental toughness.

She came to the starting lines of her early season races buzzing with energy, brimming with confidence, and fully ready to perform. And she's killing it, sweeping up the field like a maniacal Merry Maid. Her reward for laying that enormous foundation has been reaching her highest peak, one that ultimately gives her a bird's-eye view of the world from the podium's top box. She'll rip through this season. Then after the final race, she'll rack her bike and pick up her skis for a couple of months, because that's how Cheryl—who at 43 has been a pro in this game for many years— stays so damn fast year after year. She lets herself occasionally slow down.

ROLLING LIKE THE TIDES

Coaches employ periodization—not just over one season, but over many seasons, because speed is meant to ebb and flow rather than stay constant. The only way to be really fast when you want to be is to allow yourself to be slow when you don't need to be so quick. Just as the easy weeks in the Get Fast! plans allow your hard training to settle in before you build again, an easy month or two at the end of the season allows your mind and body to fully heal and reset. When you come back, you're not starting from zero, but from a higher place because you've been progressively and patiently building and repairing over time.

Taking a few steps back also helps you avoid getting caught in what I call "speed traps," where being fast becomes an all-consuming concern. I know people who have stopped racing (even though they really want to race) because they're not as fast as they know they could be. They have expectations; and worse, they are worried about other people's expectations. They're afraid to fail. They stop loving the sport because the pressure to perform is crushing their enjoyment of it. I've ventured into that territory myself. It's a terrible place to be.

Instead, think of your fitness as an ocean: vast, wide, and ever changing. Your peaks of speed are like high tide. Paddle out to catch those big waves when they come, and ride them with all you've got, enjoying the thrill and the rush and the heady intoxication that builds as the miles per hour tick into uncharted territories. When the final wave crashes to the shore, coast to a stop, and lay your bike down. Let the tides roll back to sea, and find a blanket to lie on and soak in the sun. Go buy yourself an ice cream, maybe even a double dip. Stroll. Spin. Take a vacation. So when you dip your toes in the water and see that first big wave start to swell, you'll be ready to ride again.

INDEX

Boldface page references indicate photographs. <u>Underscored</u> references indicate boxed text or charts.

A

A2 Wind Tunnel facility, 30
Accessories for increasing speed, 216–17.
    See also Bikes
Acetylcholine, 188
Achilles tendon problems, 46
Acid Check (supplement), 158
Adair, Dominique, 109–11
Adaptogens, 156–57
Adductor foam roller work, 71, 75, **75**
Adenosine, 187
Adrenaline, 190
Aerodynamic clothing, 31
Aerodynamic drag, 29, 31, 204, 210
Aerodynamic part swaps, 29
Aerodynamics, 28–30, 215. *See also* Wind
    speed
Aero watts, 30–31
Age, 78, 112
Air pollution, avoiding, 42
Air temperature, 191, 209–10
Alcohol, <u>148–49</u>, 189
Alka-Myte (supplement), 158
Allen, Hunter, 90–92, 94, <u>99</u>
Alloy handlebars, 219
Alpha-linolenic acid, 192
Aluminum bike frames, 199–200
Aluminum wheels, 216
Amino acids, 128, 152–53
Amino Vital (supplement), 156
Anabolic state, 140–41
Anaerobic thresholds, 156
Angles of bike frame, 202
Ankle strengthening, 47
Ankling, 6, 46
Annesi, Jim, 180
Applegate, Andy, 17
Apps, calorie-counting and exercise-
    tracking, 114, 147
Arent, Shawn, 155
Arginine, 156
Armstrong, Lance, 8, 52, 57, 81–82, 96
Artificial sweeteners, 128
Ascending
    back muscles and, 21
    energy and, 18
    feet position and, 20
    gear shifting and, 19–20
    Get Fast! Hill Climb Plan and, 253,
        <u>253–55</u>
    goal-setting and, 20–21
    grades, various, 21–22
    importance of doing well, 16–17
    intensity, finding ideal, 20
    interval training for more power while,
        257–58
    lactate threshold and, 20
    positive self-talk and, 167–68
    qigong climbing and, 18
    sitting and spinning, 18–19
    with speed, 16–22
Atkinson, Michael, 172

B

Back muscles, 21, 56, 74, **74**
Banting, K., 177
Basal metabolism, 111–13, 113
Basal metabolism rate (BMR), 113, 113
Baseline weight, calculating, 92, 92
Baths, 235–36
BCAAs, 122, 156
Beef, grass-fed, 149
Belief in self, 176
Benardot, Dan, 126
Beta-alanine, 154, 156, 159
Beverages. *See also* Hydration
  alcoholic, 148–49, 189
  chocolate milk, 153, 237
  coffee, 149
  diet soda, 148
  green tea, 149, 155
  recovery, 153
  sports drinks, 128, 137–38, 140
  water, 149, 148–49
Bike helmets, 217
Bikes
  aerodynamic drag and, 29
  "being one with," 185–86
  bottom bracket drop of, 203
  chainstay length of, 202–3
  compliant, 200
  cost of, 196, 212
  fit of, 217
  frame materials for, 197, 199–201
  geometry of, 201–3
  leaning, on corners, 23–24
  maintaining
    cables, 210
    chain replacement, 207–8
    drivetrain, 205–8
    handlebars, 210
    resources for, 205
    speed and, 197, 204
    tires, 208–10
    washing, 210–11
  speed and
    accessories, 216–17
    aerodynamic parts, 29
    frame materials, 199–201
    geometry, 201–3
    handlebars, 219–20
    maintenance of, 197
    overview, 196–97
    pedals, 218–19
    saddles, 217–18
    technique and, 5–6
    tires, 213–15
    weight of, 198
    wheels, 212, 215–16

"stiff," 200
stock, 217
technique and, 5
upgrades to, 212–13
wheelbase of, 202
Black tea extract, 155
Blood acid/alkaline balance, 158
Blood pressure management, 154
Blood sugar levels, 128
BMR, 113, 113
Body
  build, 96, 97
  composition, 94, 95, 112
  fat, 94
  frame size, 93–94, 93, 112
  music and, 174–75
  speed training and, 225–27
  temperature, 38–39, 188, 191–92
Body composition scale, 94
Body-mind connection, 18
Body weight
  baseline, calculating, 92, 92
  body build and, 96, 97
  body composition and, 94, 95, 112
  calories in, 142
  formulas, caution about, 94
  racing versus healthy, 92
  saddles and, 218
  shifting on bike, 13–14, 26
  steps in calculating ideal cycling
    baseline weight, 92, 92
    body composition, 94, 95
    competitive weight, 96–97,
      100
    frame size, 93–94, 93
Bonci, Leslie, 145–46, 155
Bonking
  diet and, 105, 117, 126–27
  electrolyte depletion and, 105, 127, 140
  glycogen stores and, 167
  mental distress of, 190
  muscles and, 167
  Paleo-like diet in preventing, 117
  understanding, 126–27
Bottom bracket drop of bike, 203
Brain, sugar and, 116–17, 187. *See also*
    Mental training
Brake rub, 197
Braking
  body weight shifts and, 13–14
  cornering and, 23
  descending and, 14, 25–27
  emergency, 14–15
  feathering and, 13, 23
  with front brakes, 13–14
  harder and later, 2–3
  on slippery terrain, 14

Mesomorph body build, 97
Metabolism
  age and, 112
  basal, 111–13, 113
  body composition and, 112
  body frame size and, 112
  calorie-restricted diet and, 148
  catechins and, 155
  exercise before breakfast and, 149
  gender and, 112
  hormones and, 112
  lean muscles and, 81
  water intake and, 149
MHR, 230–31, 231
Microadjustments, making, 33–34
Mifflin-St. Jeor equation, 113, 113
Milk, chocolate, 153, 237
Mind-body connection, 18
Mind, power of, 163. *See also* Mental
    training
Mini goals, 180
Mood, monitoring and controlling, 167–68,
    183–84
Motivation
  celebrating performance gains, 185
  coaches, 184–85
  controlled, 177
  flow state, finding, 185–86
  goal-setting and, 179–80
  groups rides, 181–82
  intrinsic, 177
  moods, monitoring, 183–84
  music, 184
  planning rides, 180–81
  for speed, increasing, 178
  variety to rides, adding, 182–83
Mountain biking
  cleat position and, 38
  cornering and, 23
  handlebar width and, 219
  for pedaling technique, smooth, 8
  tire width and, 214
  wax lubes and, 207
Muscles. *See also specific type*
  age and, 78
  black tea extract and, 155
  body build and, 97
  bonking and, 167
  chocolate milk and, 237
  compression clothing and, 43
  in core, 54–55
  electrolytes and, 126–27
  fast-twitch fibers, 80, 227
  human growth hormone and, 188
  hypertrophy, 78–79
  interval training for, 256–57
  massaging, 70, 238

  metabolism and lean, 81
  music and, 36, 175
  nitrogen and, 158
  plyometrics and, 80–81
  slow-twitch fibers, 227
  speed training and, 226–27
Music
  body and, 174–75
  contentions about, 44, 175
  exercise effort and, 175–76, 176
  in fatigue prevention, 165, 174–75
  lactate levels and, 36
  mental training and, 165–66, 174–76, 176
  for motivation, 184
  muscles and, 36, 175
  nervous system and, 175
  in performance improvements, 44, 165
  training and, 44

N

Narrow riding position, 30–32
Negative self-talk, 166–68
Nervous system and music, 175
Nitric oxide (NO) system, 156
Nitrogen, 158
Noakes, Timothy, 126, 167
Noise and sleep, 189
Non-REM sleep, 189
NormaTec MVP Recovery System, 239
NO system, 156
Nunn sports drink tablets, 128
Nutrition, 104–6. *See also* Diet

O

Obesity crisis, 114
Off-season, 83, 259–60
Omega-3 fatty acids, 125, 154–55, 192
OptygenHP, 154, 156–57
Organic food, 149
Overcooking a turn, avoiding, 22
Overend, Ned, 10
Oxidative stress, reducing, 155
Oxygen consumption, 18, 40. *See also*
    Energy

P

Paceline, keeping, 33–34
Pain, 54–55, 170–72
Pain threshold, 170
Paleo-like diet, 117–18
Pants, compression, 43
PAP, 46
Park, Peter, 82
Pasta, 104, 121

pedaling, 46–47
precooling body, 38–39
steering with "third eye," 2–3
sunglasses, 44–45, 45
sunscreen, 47
warmup, 45–46
tire pressure and, 209
training
body and, 225–27
breath analyzer and, 228–29
efficiency and, 227
efforts and, measuring, 228, 232–33
heart and, 226
heart rate and, 225
heart rate monitor and, 229–31, 231
intervals, 233–34
lactate levels and, 226
muscles and, 226–27
power meter and, 232
recovery from, 235–39
understanding, 225
zones for, 234, 234
"traps," 260
SPF protection, 47
Spices, 148
Spokes, 215
SportLegs (supplement), 157–58
Sports drinks, 128, 137–38, 140
Sports drink tablets, 128
Sports nutrition science, 105. See also Diet
Sprinting and cleat position, 38
Sprinting interval training, 257
Staleness, avoiding, 183–84
Stamstad, John, 170
Standing, benefits of, 76–77
Starch, 116–17, 145
Steady intervals, 233, 234
Steel bike frames, 200–201
Steering, 2–3, 24
"Stiff" bikes, 200
Strength training, traditional, 78–79, 81
Suffering, 170–72, 222–23
Sugar
brain and, 116–17, 187
in chocolate milk, 153
in pasta, 116
simple, 136
sports drinks and, adding to, 128
Sunglasses, 44–45, 45
Sunscreen, 47
Supplements
Acid Check, 158
Alka-Myte, 158
Amino Vital, 156
arginine, 156
beta-alanine, 154, 156, 159
caffeine, 158–59

creatine powder, 152
ephedra, 152
ergogenic aids, 151–52
5-Hour Energy shots, 159
money spent on sports, 151
omega-3 fatty acids, 154–55
OptygenHP, 154, 156–57
in past, 151–52
SportLegs, 157–58
tea extracts, 155
Track Stack, 159
training and, 106
whey protein, 152–53
Surfaces, cycling. See Terrain
Swain, D.P., 16
Swimming, 41–42

T

Tanita body composition scale, 94
Tea, 149
Tea extracts, 155
Technique. See also specific type
bikes and speed and, 5
braking, 13–15
breathing, 40–42
cornering, 22–24
gear shifting, 10–12
pedaling, 7, 8
speed and, 2–5
Teig, Donald, 45
Temperature. See Air temperature; Body
Tempo intervals, 233, 234
Terrain
rough, 8, 14, 209
slippery, 14
wet, 14, 209
Terry, Peter, 167–68
Thermic effect of activity, 112
Thermic effect of food, 112, 145
"Third eye," 2–3
Thirst, 129, 140, 148
Thompson, Kevin, 163
Time trials
cleat position and, 38
interval training, 250, 250–52
Tipping point, 25
Tires
maintaining, 208–10
pinch flatting and, 209
pressure of, 208–10
speed and, 213–15
thread count of, 213
tread patterns of, 214
tubeless, 214–15
tubular, 214
width of, 214